PEDIATRIC ANESTHESIA REVIEW
JUST THE FACTS

Ellen Roark Basile, DO
Pediatric Anesthesiologist
Oklahoma City, OK

S. Nini Malayaman, MD
Anesthesiologist
Drexel University College of Medicine
Philadelphia, PA

Jeremy Almon, MD
Anesthesiologist
Integris Baptist Medical Center
Oklahoma City, Ok

Tyler Kloven, DO
Clinical Anesthesiology Resident
Oklahoma City, OK

Cover Design: Nabil Aounallah, MD
Cover: Kinsley Mae Almon

Copyright © 2016 by Basile, Malayaman, Almon, and Kloven

Dedication

"I will reverence my master who taught me the art."
Hippocratic Oath, 5th Century BC

To that end, I wish to thank my masters:

Jack B. Cohen, MD
John Archer, MD
Inger Aliason, MD

Basile, DO

Contents

1. Pediatric Anesthesia - General Facts 7
2. Neonatal - General Facts 17
3. Respiratory Topics 23
4. Congenital Cardiac Topics 31
5. Common Syndromes/Congenital Anomalies 39
6. Pediatric Advanced Life Support 49
7. Malignant Hyperthermia 55
8. Regional Anesthesia/Pain 61
9. Neurosurgery Topics 69
10. Ear/Nose/Throat Topics 75
11. Pharmacology 81
12. Questions 91
13. Answers with Explanations 125
14. Sources Consulted/ References 163

Chapter 1: Pediatric Anesthesia – General Facts

- ❖ MAC
- ❖ Mapleson Circuits
- ❖ Heat Loss in Pediatric Population
- ❖ ETT Size/Depth
- ❖ Airway Differences
- ❖ NPO Guidelines
- ❖ Rapid Induction in Infants
- ❖ Induction Differences
- ❖ Anesthetics: Metabolism in Pediatrics
- ❖ Neuromuscular Receptors
- ❖ Fluid Therapy
- ❖ Estimated Blood Volumes
- ❖ Volume of Distribution
- ❖ Percent Body Mass Index
- ❖ Aspiration Risks
- ❖ Dentition
- ❖ Emergence Delirium

MAC

- Minimum alveolar concentration = potency of an inhaled anesthetic agent
- Highest MAC at 6 months old
- Progressive decrease in MAC > 6 months old
    - 6% decrease in MAC/decade
- Neonate has significantly decreased MAC
- Premature infants have even greater reduction in MAC
- Cerebral palsy/mental retardation reduce MAC 25%

Mapleson Circuits

- A   Magill
- B
- C   Waters
- D   Bain circuit
- E   Ayre's T-piece
- F   Jackson-Rees modification
- Primary differences between circuits:
    - locations of the fresh gas flow
    - location of the pop-off (relief) valve

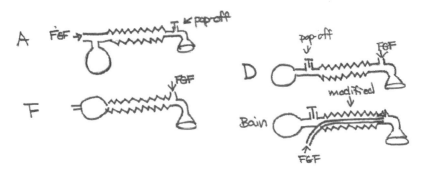

Mapleson Circuits Continued

- CO_2 retention determines suitability of circuit: spontaneous vs positive pressure ventilation
- CO_2 retention determined by the following:
  - **#1 - Fresh gas flow (FGF)**
  - Minute ventilation
  - Spontaneous (SV) vs positive pressure ventilation (PPV)
  - Tidal volume
  - Respiratory rate
  - I:E ratio
  - Peak inspiratory flow rate
- Best for spontaneous ventilation = A > DEF > BC
- Best for positive pressure ventilation = DEF > BC > A
- Please note circuits that are superior for PPV:
  - Have FGF close to the patient (mask)
  - Allow expired breath (CO_2-rich gas) to be pushed away from patient

Mapleson Advantages	Mapleson Disadvantages
Low resistance decreases work of breathing	Loss of heat
Portable	Significant pollution
No valves	High FGF requirements
Decreased volume circuit	
Decreased compression volume	

Mapleson D (Bain Circuit)

- Bain modification
  - Co-axial system
  - Fresh gas flow (FGF) enters via a tube inside of an outer tube
- Counter current principle: exhaled air (outer tube) warms inspired air (inner tube)
- Retains heat/ humidity
- Issues: possible kinking of inner tube
- Recommended FGF spontaneous ventilation = 2 – 3X minute ventilation

Mapleson E/F

- Mapleson E = Ayre's T-piece (1937)
- Mapleson F is a modified E circuit
- Mapleson F = Jackson-Rees = modified Ayre's T-piece (1950)
  - Added an open-ended breathing bag
  - Allows scavenging
- Recommended FGF spontaneous ventilation = 2 – 3X minute ventilation

Heat Loss In Pediatric Population

- Immature thermal control in infants; babies get cold really fast
- Increased body surface area: body weight ratio
- Decreased subcutaneous fat
- Increased skin permeability (thin skin)
- 90% of metabolic heat lost via skin

Operating Room Concerns

- 1 – 2° loss during 1st hour in OR
  - Redistribution from core → periphery
- **RADIATION = 40%**
  - **Primary source of heat loss in OR**
  - Heat transfer object to object, mass important
  - How the sun heats the earth
- Convection = 30%, wind chill
- Evaporative = 10%, increased in pediatrics (2° increased V_A, increased RR)
- Conduction = 5%, skin contact

Keep 'Em Warm

- WARM ROOM = most effective method (reduces radiation loss)
- 1°C increase in ambient temp decreases heat loss 7%
- Options: Bair hugger, warm mattress, fluid warmer (Hotline/Ranger)
- Cover infants head (18% BSA vs 9% BSA in adult)

Brown Fat

- Infants do not shiver
- Heat production occurs via metabolism of brown fat
- Term infant 2 – 6% brown fat (scapula, mediastinum, kidney/adrenals)
- Metabolism of brown fat requires increased oxygen consumption (VO_2) as well as increased glucose use
- Decreased amount brown fat in preemies, and sick neonates
- Volatile anesthetics inhibit brown fat metabolism

ETT Size/Depth

- Formula:
  - ETT size
    - For uncuffed ETT: Size (mm ID) = (age in years/4) + 4
    - For cuffed ETT: Size (mm ID) = (age in years/4) + 3
  - Insertion depth = ETT size × 3
- Cuffed vs uncuffed ETT
  - Most pediatric anesthesiologists routinely use cuffed ETT
  - Concern with cuffed tubes is iatrogenic airway edema
  - Increased risk for infants who are intubated for a long duration; however edema can happen in short cases if cuff pressure is too high, ETT too large, or trauma during insertion
  - Subglottic stenosis- potential consequence prolonged intubation
- Check airway leak: if no leak @ 20 cm H_2O = too tight a fit
- Recommended that cuff pressure not exceed 20 cm H_2O

*ID = internal diameter

Airway Differences

- Large occiput, short neck, large tongue
- **Larynx @ C3 – 4, glottis @ C4**
- Anterior cords
- "Floppy epiglottis", epiglottis narrow/omega-shaped
- Funnel shaped airway (infant) vs cylinder (adult)
- Cricoid ring considered narrowest portion of airway in infants
  - vs rima glottis in adults
  - Until approximately 8 years old

NPO Guidelines

Ingested Material	Minimum Fasting Period
Clear liquids	2 h
Breast milk	4 h
Infant formula/G-tube	6 h
Nonhuman milk	6 h
Light meal	6 h
Heavy meal (fat/protein)	8 h

These recommendations apply to healthy patients undergoing elective procedures

Rapid Induction in Infants

- Explanations for rapid inhalation mask induction in infants
    - **Increased V_A : FRC**   *most important*
        - **Alveolar ventilation: functional residual capacity ratio**
    - Altered distribution of cardiac output
    - Decreased blood: gas solubility in infants
    - Decreased tissue: blood solubility

Induction Differences in Infants

- V_A: FRC ratio
    - Adult 1.5 : 1 vs **Pediatric 5 : 1**
    - V_A = Alveolar Ventilation = (Tidal Vol – Dead Space) × RR
    - V_A increased secondary to increased RR in infants
    - FRC = Functional Residual Capacity = (Exp Reserve Volume + Residual Volume)
- Cardiac Output
    - Infant 22% CO to vessel rich group (brain, heart)
    - Adult 10% CO to vessel rich group
- Blood solubility of inhalation agents are decreased 18% in neonates
    - Secondary to decreased serum cholesterol and proteins
    - Recall: decreased solubility = increased rate of onset
- Tissue/gas solubility is ½ that of adults
    - Secondary to increased H_2O content and decreased protein

Anesthetics: Metabolism in Pediatrics

- Liver has decreased function @ birth
    - Phase I reaction = oxidation/reduction
    - Phase II reaction = conjugation
    - Multiple Cytochrome P450 enzymes not fully functioning at birth
    - **Decreased metabolism increases medication half-life**
- Protein binding
    - Neonates ↓ albumin concentration (adult levels at 5 months)
    - **↓ protein binding = ↑ free drug**
        - Albumin has decrease binding capacity
        - Neonates plasma has substances that reduce protein binding: bilirubin, maternal steroids
- Excretion
    - Kidney receives
        - 5 – 6% cardiac output neonate
        - 20 – 25% cardiac output adult
    - GFR term infant 40% of adult
    - GFR preemie 20 – 30% of adult
    - **Decreased GFR delays drug elimination**
    - Decreased ability to concentrate urine
    - Potassium levels are naturally elevated in neonates, and young infants

Neuromuscular Receptors

- Adult nicotinic receptor (mature): 2α, β, d, Σ **(epsilon)**
    - Located at neuromuscular endplate
    - Shorter mean opening duration
- Fetal nicotinic receptor (immature): 2α, β, d, γ **(gamma)**
    - Located at neuromuscular endplates as well as throughout muscle
    - 10-fold increase in opening duration (Na^+ goes in, K^+ flows out)
- Immature nicotinic receptors will repopulate after injury:
    - Denervation, burns, immobilization
- α subunit is binding unit for ACh and NMBDs
- Rocuronium has increased onset in infants, increased potency, and decreased clearance
    - Potency: infants >> adults
- Prolonged muscle relaxation: hypothermia, antibiotics, renal failure, age (infancy)

Fluid Therapy

- Need to know weight of pt. Below are approximate estimates
    - 1 year old ~ 10 kg
    - 2 year old ~ 12 kg
    - 3 year old ~ 14 kg
    - 4 year old ~ 16 kg
    - 5 year old ~ 20 kg
  ***there can be wide individual variances from these estimates

- To calculate maintenance fluids/hour = patient's weight × fluid volume as listed:

Weight (kg)	Fluid (volume ml/kg/hr)
<10	4
10 – 20	40 ml for 1st 10 kg + 2 ml/kg
>20	60 ml for 1st 20 kg + 1 ml/kg

- Fluid deficit = maintenance fluids per hour × NPO hours*
- Consider limiting hours of NPO to avoid volume overloading (i.e. 8 hrs NPO)

Estimated Blood Volumes

- Premature neonate   95 – 100 ml/kg
- Term infant   85 ml/kg
- Infant 1 yr old   80 ml/kg
- Adult male   75 ml/kg
- Adult female   65 ml/kg
- Pregnant female   100 ml/kg

Volume of Distribution

- Infants have increased volume of distribution (V_D)
- Total body water
    - 70% TBW infants vs 60% TBW adults
    - Increased **extracellular compartment** is primarily responsible
    - Increased V_D = increased intubating dose, however ↓ maintenance dose needed

Percent (%) Body Mass Index

	NEWBORN	ADULT
Vessel-rich group	22	10
Muscle	38	50
Fat	13	22

Aspiration Risks

- 10X > for emergency cases vs elective cases
- Neurologic or esophagogastric abnormality
- ASA physical status class 3 – 5
- Increased intracranial pressure
- Increased abdominal pressure (pregnancy, bowel obstruction)
- More likely to occur at induction than at emergence
- <3 year old

Dentition
- Primary/deciduous/"baby" teeth
    - Total number = 20 (10 upper, 10 lower)
    - Usually, two bottom front teeth emerge first at 6 – 10 months old
    - Top four teeth emerge at 8-12 months
    - By 2-3 years old, all primary teeth should be present
- Secondary/permanent teeth
    - Total number = 32 (16 upper, 16 lower)
    - Emerge when primary teeth are lost at 6 – 11 years old
- Any loose teeth? Make inquiry, most commonly lost between 5 – 7 years old

Emergence Delirium

- Definition = dissociated state of consciousness, patient is inconsolable, psychomotor agitation, combative, thrashing, does not appear to be coherent but is awake - You'll know it when you see it!
- Highest incidence: pre-school age children, 2 – 5 years old
- Triggers: volatile anesthetic – sevoflurane> isoflurane > halothane
- Possible triggers: midazolam, ketamine
- Related surgeries???
    - ENT: tonsils, thyroid, middle ear
    - Eye
- Behavior is usually self-limiting
- Possible treatment
    - Opioids
    - Dark, quiet room
    - Propofol
    - Midazolam?????? No
- There is no known definitive treatment, almost everything has been tried with marginal results
- *Clinically, we have found a small bolus of Propofol (0.3 – 0.5mg/kg) is enough to put patient back to sleep extremely effective; reset the clock, so to speak*
- *Of note, if you have a patient with known emergence delirium, try GA with TIVA (propofol infusion)*

Chapter 2: Neonatal - General Facts

- ❖ Definitions
- ❖ APGAR Score
- ❖ Respiratory Distress Syndrome
- ❖ Apnea of Prematurity
- ❖ Umbilical Cord vs Adult ABG
- ❖ Hemoglobin F vs Hemoglobin A
- ❖ Physiologic Anemia
- ❖ Meconium Aspiration
- ❖ Post-Gestational Age
- ❖ Intraventricular Hemorrhage (IVH)
- ❖ EXIT procedure

Definitions

- Premature/Preterm = infants born <37 weeks gestation
- Term infant = 37 – 42 weeks gestation
- Post term = >42 weeks gestation
- Low birth weight = <2500 gm
- Very low birth weight = <1500 gm
- Micro preemie = <750 gm
- Infant = less than one year old
- Neonate = less than one month old

APGAR Score

	0	1	2	Total Points
Activity	Absent	Arms/legs flexed	Active	
Pulse	Absent	<100 BPM	>100 BPM	
Grimace (reflex)	Flaccid	Some flexion	Sneeze/ cough	
Appearance	Blue pale	*Pink torso/ hands feet blue	Completely pink	
Respiration	Absent	Slow, irregular	Vigorous cry	

- Total Points:
    - 0 – 3 = Severe depression
    - 4 – 6 = Moderate depression
    - 7 – 10 = Excellent condition
- Virginia Apgar, MD – anesthesiologist
- APGAR number indicates level of asphyxia in newborn
- Consider APGAR a point of care test
    - i.e. measurement of patient's condition at that exact moment in time
- APGAR is NOT a predictor of mortality and morbidity
- *Acrocyanosis = pink torso with blue extremities (hands/ feet)

Respiratory Distress Syndrome (RDS)

- RDS = hyaline membrane disease, surfactant deficiency
- Decreased surfactant = alveolar collapse = atelectasis
    - Atelectasis results in shunting of blood (shunt = perfusion without ventilation)
- Disease of prematurity
- Signs/symptoms: grunting, nasal flaring, chest retractions, tachypnea
- Treatment: PEEP + exogenous surfactant

Apnea of Prematurity

- Apnea = cessation of breathing for 20 seconds
- **Post-gestational age is inversely related to apnea risk**
- Additional risk factors for apnea of prematurity:
    - HCT <30% = increased risk
    - Type of surgery
    - Infant <36 weeks gestation at birth
- Recommended: former preterm infant <55 – 60 weeks post-gestational age
    - Admit post-op for observation
    - Monitor for at least 12 apnea-free hours
- Regional vs GA: no difference in post-op apnea
- Caffeine base 10 mg/ml IV or caffeine citrate 20 mg/ml IV
    - Used as treatment in NICU

Umbilical Cord Blood vs Adult ABG

	pH	pCO_2	pO_2	HCO_3
Umbilical artery	7.28	49	18	22
Umbilical vein	7.35	38	29	20
Adult FiO_2 21%	7.4	35	95 – 100	24

Hemoglobin F vs Hemoglobin A

- Hemoglobin F = Fetal hemoglobin
- Hemoglobin F = α_2, γ_2 (2 alpha, 2 gamma)
- Hemoglobin A = α_2, β_2 (2 alpha, 2 beta)
- O_2-Hb curve shifted left for Hb F
    - Hb F p50 at 19 mmHg O_2
    - Hb A p50 at 26 mmHg O_2
- 2,3-diphosphoglycerate (2,3-DPG) binds β (beta) subunit in Hb A
    - 2,3-DPG changes shape of molecule, enables unloading of O_2 from Hb
    - Increased 2,3-DPG decreases O_2 affinity for the Hb molecule
- Hb F does not have a beta subunit, resulting in left-shifted O_2-Hb curve, increased O_2 affinity
- Hydroxyurea = Rx commonly used in sickle cell disease, increases level of Hb F

Physiological Anemia

- Natural physiologic process
- Decreased erythropoiesis, transitioning hemoglobin F to hemoglobin A
- At birth hemoglobin 18 – 19 g/dL, hematocrit 60%
    - Hemoglobin F 80% at term
- Anemia nadir term infant at 8 – 12 weeks of life, hemoglobin 11 g/dL
- Anemia nadir premature infant at 7 – 10 weeks of life, hemoglobin <11 g/dL

Meconium Aspiration

- Meconium = fecal matter made by fetus in utero
- Fetal hypoxia secondary to aspiration of meconium
- Persistent pulmonary hypertension
    - May require ECMO (extracorporeal membrane oxygenation)
- Respiratory failure
- Interventions at birth if meconium staining or frank aspiration:
    - Routine suctioning of oropharynx
    - If newborn vigorous and crying, do not intubate
    - If newborn depressed
        - Intubate
        - Suction endotracheal tube
        - If bradycardia present, provide positive pressure ventilation

Post-Gestational Age

- A calculation of infant's time since conception
- **Post-gestational age (PGA) = weeks in utero at delivery + weeks alive since delivery**
    - Used as a guide by pediatric anesthesiologists when taking care of premature infants to predict possible post-operative apnea, possible need for additional post-op monitoring and/or admission
- Most pediatric hospitals have written policies regarding post-op observation
    - 55 – 60 weeks post gestational age will generally require overnight admission
- **Corrected age = number of weeks alive - number of weeks premature**
    - Corrected age is a completely different calculation
    - Used as a guide by pediatricians for anticipated delays in milestones and development
    - Example: 6-months-old infant born 12 weeks premature
        Corrected age = 24 weeks alive - 12 weeks premature
        = 12 weeks old = 3 months old

Intraventricular Hemorrhage (IVH)

- Disease of prematurity
- Diagnosis: ultrasound
- Primary site venous-capillary connection
- Gestational age inversely related to risks of developing IVH
    - Grade I = subependymal bleed, no IVH
    - Grade II = +IVH, no ventricular dilation
    - Grade III = +IVH with mild ventricular dilation
    - Grade IV = +IVH with ventricular dilation, and parenchymal blood
- Grades III and IV have poor neurological outcomes

EXIT procedure

- EXIT = **EX** utero **I**ntrapartum **T**reatment
- Performed at the time of caesarean section
- Indications:
    - Airway control - most common reason for EXIT procedure
        - Most common airway anomaly requiring EXIT = cervical teratoma
    - ECMO - for severe congenital cardiac condition
    - Resection of high-risk tumor
    - Separation (conjoined twins)
- Fetal concerns
    - **Fetus delivered via laparotomy with umbilical perfusion maintained**
    - Anesthetize with fentanyl, atropine, muscle relaxant
    - Airway secured by ENT surgeon - ETT vs tracheostomy
    - Monitored: pulse oximetry and echocardiography
- Maternal concerns
    - General anesthesia with RSI induction
    - Uterine relaxation paramount
        - High inspired volatile anesthetic
        - Nitroglycerine
    - Left lateral position for uterine displacement
- Once fetal airway is secured
    - Umbilical cord clamped
    - Uterine relaxation reversed
- Increased maternal risks
    - Hemorrhage
    - Wound healing

Chapter 3: Respiratory Topics

- ❖ Development
- ❖ Surfactant
- ❖ Pulmonary Facts
- ❖ Lung Volumes
- ❖ Upper Respiratory Infection
- ❖ Obstructive/Restrictive Lung Disease
- ❖ Asthma
- ❖ Bronchopulmonary Dysplasia
- ❖ Congenital Lung Abnormalities
- ❖ Cystic Fibrosis
- ❖ Mediastinal Mass

Development

- Early development
    - In utero (week)
    - Week 4: Lung buds
    - Week 5: Bronchial buds
    - Week 5: Primary bronchi (2 left, 3 right)
    - Week 5 – 17: Pseudoglandular period
        - Respiration not possible
    - Week 13 – 28: Canalicular period
        - Respiratory bronchioles & terminal sacs
    - Week 24 – Birth: Terminal sac period
        - Cell differentiation occurs:
            - Two types of pneumocytes
            - Type 1 = gas exchange (O_2, CO_2), 90% alveolar surface
            - Type 2 = surfactant, 10% alveolar surface
    - Week 29 – 8 years old: Alveolar period
- Lung development continues after birth until age 8 – 10 years
- # of alveoli
    - Infants: 24 million
    - Adults: 300 million
- CXR: Newborn lung denser than adults secondary to decreased number of alveoli

Surfactant

- Type II pneumocytes = alveolar epithelial cells
    - Can reproduce, unlike type 1 pneumocytes
- Surfactant contains:
    - Phospholipids
    - Proteins
    - Ions
    - Calcium
- Phospholipids = hydrophilic & hydrophobic end
    - Hydrophobic end = 1/12 to ½ surface tension of H_2O
- **Surfactant decreases surface tension of alveoli, which keeps alveoli open**
- Laplace's Law:

$$P = 2T/r$$

P is the pressure (dyne/cm)
T is the surface tension (dyne cm^2)
r is the radius (cm)

Pulmonary Facts

- Physiologic shunt fraction neonate 10 – 20% compared to adult 2 – 5%
- Aa gradient neonate > adult
- Diaphragm
    - Type 1 fibers = slow twitch, **resist fatigue**, high oxidative
        - Muscle composition slow twitch fibers %:
        - Fetal 10%, term 25%, adult 55%
        - Explanation for early respiratory fatigue in neonates
    - Type II fibers = fast twitch, strength, fatigue easily
- **Neonatal lungs = LESS COMPLIANT**
- Increased airway resistance:
    - Decreased elastin = airway more likely to collapse, elastin allows for recoil
    - Diameter of alveolar bronchi, respiratory bronchi important
    - Poiseuille's equation $\Delta P = \dfrac{8\mu L Q}{\pi r^4}$

        or

        $R \, \alpha \, \dfrac{L \times viscocity}{r4}$

        P = Pressure
        R = Resistance
        μ = dynamic viscosity
        Q = volumetric flow rate
        L = length of pipe
        r = radius

- Chest wall = INCREASED COMPLIANCE
    - Pediatric ribs are more cartilaginous rather than bone, which allows greater movement, i.e. collapse

        $compliance = \dfrac{\Delta Volume}{\Delta Pressure}$

Lung Volumes

- Infant same as adult:
    - Tidal volume: 5 – 7 ml/kg
    - Functional residual capacity (FRC): 27 – 30 ml/kg
    - Dead space: 2-2.5 ml/kg
- Infant greater than adult
    - Alveolar ventilation (V_A): **Infant 100 – 150 ml/kg/min**
        Adult 60 ml/kg/min
    - O_2 consumption: **Infant 6 – 8 ml/kg/min**
        Adult 3 ml/kg/min

Upper Respiratory Infection (URI)

- **DANGER, CAUTION, proceed with great care**
- Reasons to possibly cancel "elective" case:
    - >38.5 °C, fever indicates systemic response, infection likely
    - Lethargic, droopy, poor PO intake
    - Active wheezing
    - Signs of lower respiratory tract infection
        - Cough, rales, rhonchi
        - Yellow, green sputum
- Airway can remain reactive 4 – 6 weeks s/p URI
- **Anticipate increased airway reactivity in patients <2 years old with URI**
- **↑↑↑ Increased risk airway compromise: laryngospasm, bronchospasm**

Obstructive/Restrictive Lung Disease

Obstructive	Restrictive
Asthma	Interstitial lung disease
Bronchiolitis	Neuromuscular disease
Cystic fibrosis	Scoliosis
Emphysema	Tuberculosis

- Obstructive lung disease = resistance to air flow
    - Predominantly effects exhalation
    - Air trapping
    - FEV_1/FVC <70%
    - INCREASED lung volumes: residual volume and total lung capacity
    - V/Q mismatch
- Restrictive lung disease = decreased compliance
    - Increased work of breathing
    - DECREASED lung volumes as well as lung capacities
    - Normal FEV_1/FVC

Asthma

- M > F in children <15 year old
- Most common chronic disease in children in developed countries
- Precipitating factors
    - Upper respiratory infection
    - Allergic reaction
    - Mechanical stimulation (ETT)
    - Environmental - allergies/seasonal
    - Emotional stress
    - Exercise
- Bronchospasm = airway obstruction
- Peripheral airways > proximal
- Cholinergic Receptors: acetylcholine = bronchoconstriction
- Increased dead space secondary to air trapping
    - CO_2 predominately affected
        - Increased RV, FRC, TLC
        - Decreased VC, ERV, IC
- Diagnosis:
    - Spirometry
        - FEV_1/FVC < 70% indicates obstructive disease
    - Post-bronchodilator pulmonary function test
        - Positive result if > 12% increase from baseline FEV_1
- Treatment:
    - Anticholinergics
        - Glycopyrrolate
        - Ipratropium solution
        - Mechanism:
            - Inhibits acetylcholine
            - Dilation of proximal airway, bronchi
            - Decreases mucous production
    - Beta 2 agonist
        - Albuterol
        - Epinephrine
        - Terbutaline
        - Mechanism
            - Beta 2 agonist
            - Smooth muscle relaxation
    - Corticosteroids
    - Methylxanthines

Bronchopulmonary Dysplasia (BPD)

- Definition: chronic lung disease
    - Need for supplemental O_2
    - Diagnosed when >28 days of life
- Highly correlated with prematurity
- Etiology:
    - Prolonged ventilation
    - Supplemental O_2
    - Infection
- Treatment: bronchodilators, +/- furosemide (Lasix)
- **CO_2 retention leads to compensatory metabolic alkalosis**
- Furosemide adverse effects:
    - Hypernatremia
    - Decreased K^+, Ca^{2+} and Cl^-
    - Metabolic alkalosis

Congenital Lung Abnormalities

- **Congenital cystic adenomatoid malformation (CCAM)** = lack of normal alveoli, cystic dilation in terminal bronchioles
    - No gas exchange
    - Most receive pulmonary artery blood flow
    - Risks: infection, spontaneous pneumothorax
    - Treatment: surgical resection, lobectomy, may be candidate for fetal surgery/EXIT procedure
- **Lobar emphysema** = intrinsic defect bronchial cartilage = airway collapse = air trapping
    - Left upper lobe most common
    - Clinical Si/Sx: respiratory distress, CXR = hyperinflation, mediastinal shift
    - Treatment: surgical resection, avoid overexpansion of lung
- **Bronchopulmonary sequestration** = abnormal, non-functioning lung tissue
    - Does not communicate with tracheobronchial tree
    - Most often lower lobes
    - **Arterial** blood supply from aorta
    - AV fistula possible

Cystic Fibrosis

- Chronic respiratory disease
- 1:2,500 incidence
- Autosomal recessive, chromosome #7
- Disease of exocrine glands, altered electrolyte content, Cl^- channel
- Organ systems affected
    - Pulmonary = most common
        - 90% of CF patients have pulmonary complications
    - GI
    - Vas deferens absent (male sterility)
    - Nasal/mucous membranes
- Pulmonary
    - Frequent respiratory infections, chronic obstruction
    - S. aureus, H. influenzae, Pseudomonas
    - Destruction of lung tissue leads to fibrosis
    - Obstructive respiratory physiology, increased FRC, decreased FEV_1
    - PaO_2 affected > CO_2
    - Chronic antibiotics
    - Nebulized hypertonic 7% NS accelerates mucous clearance
- GI
    - Pancreatic insufficiency
    - Malnutrition
    - Insulin-dependent DM
    - Biliary cirrhosis
    - Bowel obstruction
    - Meconium ileus in newborn test for CF
- Cardiac
    - Cor pulmonale
- Ear Nose/Throat
    - Nasal polyps = #1 surgery for pediatric patients with CF

Mediastinal Mass

- Position of mass and likely diagnosis
    - Anterior: **LYMPHOMA**, Hodgkin, thymoma
        - **Most common in adolescents
        - **Non-Hodgkin lymphoma can double in size in 12 hrs**
    - Middle: foregut malformation
    - Posterior: neuroblastoma, ganglioneuroma
- Anterior Mediastinal Mass workup:
    - Labs: CBC, coagulation profile, type and cross
    - CT or MRI: evaluate airway
        - 50% tracheal compression = **significant risk of airway collapse**
    - ECHO: evaluate great vessels and chambers for signs of compression
    - CXR: evaluate for mass effect, pneumothorax, mediastinal shift, pleural effusions common
    - PFTs: may show obstructive and restrictive dysfunction
- Orthopnea = dyspnea with supine position
    - **Do not attempt general anesthesia without treatment**
    - Patient should receive steroids + radiation therapy prior to GA
    - Consider local anesthetic for lymph node biopsy
- Most common presenting sign: wheeze - mistaken for asthma
    - New onset wheeze check CXR
- Goals of anesthesia include:
    - Have ENT on standby
    - Have ECMO on standby
    - Maintain spontaneous ventilation
    - Avoid muscle relaxation due to **risk of airway collapse**
    - Lateral or prone position to relieve mass effect

ABILITY TO INTUBATE PATIENT DOES NOT ENSURE ABILITY TO VENTILATE PATIENT
This is about as serious as it gets for anesthesia

Chapter 4: Congenital Cardiac Topics

- ❖ Cardiac Development
- ❖ Fetal Circulation
- ❖ Neonatal Heart
- ❖ Atrial Septal Defect
- ❖ Ventricular Septal Defect
- ❖ Coarctation of Aorta
- ❖ Tetralogy of Fallot
- ❖ Hypoplastic Left Heart Syndrome
- ❖ Norwood/Bi-Directional Glenn/Fontan
- ❖ Patent Ductus Arteriosus
- ❖ Transposition of the Great Arteries
- ❖ Cardiopulmonary Bypass Effects
- ❖ Inhaled Nitric Oxide (iNO)
- ❖ Alpha STAT/ pH STAT

Pediatric Cardiac Anesthesia is a sub-specialty of a sub-specialty. There are LARGE textbooks devoted to this topic. This chapter will review some of the most common anomalies encountered and high-yield topics.

Cardiac Development

- Begins 3 – 8 weeks gestation
    - 2 tubes
    - 3 sections - from cephalic to caudal: bulbus cordis, ventricle, and atrium
- 22 days: cardiac loop, atria become cephalad to ventricles now caudad, heart beats
- 23 days: fusion of 2 tubes
- 26 days: septum primum appears, AV canal
- 32 days: truncus divides (aorta, pulmonary artery)
- 41 days: ostium primum closed
- 44 days: intraventricular septum closed, aortic pulmonary valves
- Fetal circulation considered "in-parallel"
    - In-parallel = both right and left ventricles provide systemic circulation
- Adult circulation considered " in-series"
    - In-series = right heart pumps to lungs, left heart provides systemic circulation sequentially

Fetal Circulation

- 1 vein = oxygenated hemoglobin: from placenta to fetus
- 2 arteries = deoxyhemoglobin: from fetus to placenta
- 3 shunts
    - **Ductus arteriosus** = artery that connects pulmonary artery to aorta
        - Oxygenated Hb bypasses lung
        - Right-to-left shunt in utero
    - **Ductus venosus** = vein that connects umbilical vein to IVC
        - Carries oxygenated Hb (70% O_2 saturation, PaO_2 30 mmHg)
        - Bypasses liver
    - **Foramen ovale** = formed by flap of septum primum between right and left atrium
        - Oxygenated Hb bypasses right ventricle and lungs via this communication
        - Right-to-left shunt in utero

Neonatal Heart

- Considered less compliant than adult heart
    - Myofibrils lack organization
    - Myocytes have decreased ability to store Ca^{2+}
- Decreased # of mitochondria (powerhouse, ATP)
- At birth, circulation coverts from parallel to series
    - Recall in utero right ventricle provides large percent of cardiac output
    - At birth, left ventricle expected to take over
        - Right heart pumps to lungs, left heart pumps to body
- 10X increase in pulmonary blood flow at birth
    - 2° to decreased pulmonary vascular resistance (PVR)
    - Breathing/oxygenation primarily responsible for decreased PVR
- Left ventricular stroke volume doubles at birth
- Patent ductus arteriosus - functional closure 1st 24 hrs of life, 2° to O_2
- Cardiac output (CO) in newborn highest of any age group
    - 200 ml/kg/min
    - 2 – 3X adult cardiac output
- Cardiac output in the neonate is rate dependent
    - CO = HR × SV
- HR is considered maximum capacity at birth

Atrial Septal Defect (ASD)

- **Acyanotic**
- Communication (hole) between right and left atrium
- Left-to-right shunt concerns:
    - Possible RA/RV overload
    - RBBB common from RV overload
    - Pulmonary congestion possible
    - Frequent pneumonias
- Si/Sx: may be completely asymptomatic
    - + murmur, mid-systolic, split S1,S2
- Several different ASD types characterized by location
    - Sinus venosus ASD = upper portion of atrial septum
    - Secundum ASD = most common, communication at region of fossa ovalis, 10 – 20% of these associated with mitral valve prolapsed (MVP), female > male
    - Ostium primum ASD = lower portion of atrial septum
- Commonly closed in cath lab with an Amplatzer septal occluder device
    - Size and location of ASD important
- For defects that cannot be closed with device, open heart surgery may be required

Ventricular Septal Defect (VSD)

- **Acyanotic**
- Most common congenital heart disease
- 3.5: 1,000 live births
- Communication(hole) between right and left ventricles
- Four common types
    - Atrioventricular canal type VSD
    - Muscular VSD
    - Perimembranous VSD = 80% of cases, most common
    - Supracristal VSD
- Left to right shunt concerns
    - pulmonary congestion
    - CHF
    - pulmonary hypertension
- Si/Sx: may present as cardiac failure
    - Dyspnea and/or sweating with feeding, tachypnea, + murmur
    - Other congenital anomalies common
- Common Rx: digoxin, furosemide (Lasix)
- Frequently require open heart surgery with CPB and patch closure
- Cath lab = possible transcatheter closure
- Post-op: pulmonary HTN, arrhythmias, and hypertension common occurrences

Coarctation of the Aorta

- **Acyanotic**
- 5% of all congenital heart disease
- Narrowing of the aorta, most frequently at the juxtaductal position (near the ductus arteriosus)
- Concerns: poor perfusion distal to coarctation, diminished/absent femoral pulses, hypertension above lesion, CHF, respiratory distress
- Si/Sx can be completely asymptomatic, or present as a critically ill neonate
- Newborns who present are usually prostaglandin dependent, and may be severely acidotic, with poor LV function
- Asymptomatic, incidental finding with HTN on upper extremities, large gradient between upper and lower extremity NIBP
- Repaired usually in first year of life, left thoracotomy, end-to-end anastomosis of aorta
- Be aware: aorta X-clamp above and below lesion during repair, bleeding, monitoring upper and lower extremity SpO_2 as well as BPs standard.

Tetralogy of Fallot

- **Cyanotic**
- Most common right-to-left shunt
- 6 – 11% of congenital heart disease
- Tetrad : VSD, overriding aorta, RV hypertrophy, right ventricular outflow tract obstruction
- TET spells = hypercyanotic spells
    - Occurs when there is a sudden decrease of oxygen in blood
- TET spell treatment goals: increase SVR, lower PVR, which should decrease shunting
    - Phenylephrine (increases SVR, lowers HR)
    - Fluid bolus (increases stroke volume)
    - Morphine (calms child thus decreasing PVR)
    - 100% O_2, hyperventilate (lowers PVR)
    - Rx: β-blockers, propranolol to relax infundibular spasm (also lowers HR)
- Ketamine considered gold standard for induction agent
- Usually repaired in infancy with open heart surgery, CPB
- Frequently will return as young adults with pulmonary stenosis requiring intervention

Hypoplastic Left Heart Syndrome

- **Cyanotic**
- 2: 10,000 live births
- Considered a single ventricle heart
- Very severe anomaly, was a fatal diagnosis prior to palliative surgery options
- Features: hypoplastic left ventricle, absent mitral valve, severe hypoplastic aorta/aortic arch
- Concerns:
    - Minimal to no cardiac output via aorta
    - Cyanosis/ hypoxia (no left side heart, no oxygenated blood to body)
    - Metabolic acidosis common (lactic acidosis from decreased perfusion)
    - Prostaglandin-dependent
        - Rely on ductus arteriosus for cardiac output to body
- Surgical options: heart transplant vs surgical palliation
- Surgical palliation: Norwood/Bi-directional Glenn/Fontan procedures

Norwood/Bi-Directional Glenn/Fontan

- A sequence of palliative open heart surgeries that result in a single ventricle responsible for cardiac output to the body
- Delivery of venous blood to the lungs is without a pump, passive drainage
- **Norwood**: 1st stage
    - Neonate
    - Procedure creates a new aorta (neo-aorta) from the pulmonary artery and existing aorta, pulmonary artery branches are disconnected from pulmonary artery trunk, systemic-pulmonary shunt created (BT shunt)
    - Very high risk surgery
- **Bi-Directional Glenn**: 2nd stage procedure
    - Performed at approximately 6 mos
    - Superior vena cava disconnected from right atrium, and connected to pulmonary artery, SVC to right PA (usually)
- **Fontan**: 3rd stage, final procedure
    - Variable time frame 3 – 5 years of age
    - Connects inferior vena cava to pulmonary artery, usually via an extra cardiac conduit.
        - Conduit may be fenestrated (communication with right atrium)
    - Concerns: Fontan patients tend to be volume dependent
        - Upper respiratory infections increase PVR and greatly effect oxygenation
        - Avoid maneuvers that increase PVR (PEEP, acidosis, hypoxia)
        - AV collaterals common, decreases oxygen saturation

Patent Ductus Arteriosus

- 10% of congenital heart disease
- In fetal circulation, ductus arteriosus provides a shunt from right heart to systemic circulation, a R-L shunt with oxygenated blood
    - High PVR is responsible for this shunt
- After birth, if ductus fails to close (with breathing/ oxygenation) shunt will typically reverse and become left to right with pulmonary over perfusion
    - SVR > PVR is responsible for the reversal of the shunt.
- Commonly associated with prematurity
- Si/Sx: bounding pulses, wide pulse pressure (low diastolic), continuous murmur "MACHINE-like", respiratory distress, oliguria
- Treatment: pharmacologic vs surgery vs cath lab
    - Rx: IV indomethacin or ibuprofen = COX-inhibitors, inhibit prostaglandin production
    - Surgery: via left thoracotomy with surgical clip closing ductus
        - Concerns: difficulty ventilating while left lung retracted for procedure, tearing of PA, clamping wrong vessel (distal aorta, common mistake), left recurrent laryngeal nerve palsy
    - Cath lab: percutaneous closure with Amplatzer duct occluder

Transposition of the Great Arteries

- **Cyanotic**
- 6% of congenital heart disease
- Aorta arises from the right ventricle, and the pulmonary artery arises from the left ventricle
    - Blood considered to be circulating in-parallel, as opposed to in-series
- Completely dependent on mixing of blood for oxygenation s/p delivery, either via ductus arteriosus, or an ASD/VSD
    - Atrial septostomy- creates a hole between right and left atrium, temporizing measure
- Coronary artery position of critical importance
- D-TGA most common type, D = dextro or right-sided,
    - Right atrium → right ventricle → aorta → body
    - Left atrium → left ventricle → pulmonary artery → lungs
- Patients are frequently prostaglandin dependent, for mixing of blood via the ductus
- Concerns: pulmonary hypertension develops early in these patients, matter of days
- Surgical repair: newborn, arterial switch procedure, requires CPB

Cardiopulmonary Bypass Effects

- SIRS = Systemic Inflammatory Response Syndrome
    - Fever >38 °C
    - Heart rate >90 or bradycardia if <1 year old
    - Respiratory rate >20
    - White blood cell # >12,000 or <4,000 with >10% bands
- Myocardial ischemia/cross clamp/reperfusion injury
    - Stiff myocardium has decreased compliance, preload important
- Air in coronaries = ST elevation, arrhythmias
- Platelet dysfunction = bleeding, coagulopathy common
- V/Q mismatch = increased A-a gradient
- Pulmonary hypertension, neonates/infants common

Inhaled Nitric Oxide (iNO)

- NOT the same as nitrous oxide (N_2O)
- Utilized for treatment of pulmonary hypertension
    - Pulmonary hypertension results in hypoxia
    - Nitric oxide produces vasodilation of pulmonary vasculature
    - Improves V/Q mismatch
- Other common uses: post cardiopulmonary bypass, congenital diaphragmatic hernia, right ventricular failure
- Delivery is via adaptation to ventilator, though can be given via face mask
- Metabolism: rapid via red blood cell, reaction with oxy-hemoglobin
- Adverse effect: produces methemoglobin, may require checking levels, abrupt withdrawal can result in rebound pulmonary hypertension

Alpha STAT vs pH STAT

- Two theories/approaches to analyze arterial blood samples during hypothermia
    - Alpha STAT and pH STAT
    - Some clinicians believe pH and $PaCO_2$ of the hypothermic blood sample should be "corrected" to reflect the patient's actual **hypothermic temperature (pH STAT)**
- Hypothermia = ↑ solubility = ↓ partial pressures of CO_2 and O_2 mmHg
    - ABG at 17 °C normal values: pH 7.6 and $PaCO_2$ 15 – 18 mmHg
    - ABG warmed to 37 °C will show higher value for PaO_2 and $PaCO_2$ and lower pH compared to that of the hypothermic patient
    - Hypothermia → hypocarbia → cerebral vasoconstriction = decreased perfusion
        - 1:1 correlation, CO_2 and cerebral vasculature
- pH STAT utilized in pediatrics for deep hypothermia, pt temp entered into ABG analyzer
    - $PaCO_2$ is maintained at 40 mmHg and the pH is maintained at 7.40 when measured at the patient's actual temperature (hypothermic)
    - CO_2 is added to oxygenator to compensate for increase solubility of CO_2 at lower temp, believed to improve cerebral perfusion
- Neurological outcomes are believe to be different mechanisms
    - Adults: thrombotic
    - Pediatrics: hypoperfusion

Alpha STAT	pH STAT
pH 7.4, $PaCO_2$ 40 when measured at 37 °C	pH 7.4, $PaCO_2$ 40 at patient's actual/cool temp
Left-shifted O_2-Hb curve	Right-shifted O_2-Hb curve
Hypocarbia	CO_2 added to oxygenator
Blood pH alkalotic when patient cooled	Blood pH neutral when patient is cool
Utilized in adult patients	Utilized in pediatric patients
Low cerebral perfusion	Increased cerebral perfusion
Allows cerebral autoregulation to function	CBF and $CMRO_2$ become uncoupled

Chapter 5: Common Syndromes/Congenital Anomalies

- ❖ CHARGE Syndrome
- ❖ VACTERL Association
- ❖ Difficult Airway Syndromes
- ❖ Congenital Diaphragmatic Hernia (CDH)
- ❖ Abdominal Defects
- ❖ Duchenne Muscular Dystrophy
- ❖ DiGeorge Syndrome
- ❖ Pyloric Stenosis
- ❖ Tracheoesophageal Fistula (TEF)
- ❖ Neuroblastoma
- ❖ Wilms Tumor
- ❖ Down Syndrome
- ❖ ECMO criteria
- ❖ TORCH Syndrome
- ❖ Scoliosis

CHARGE Syndrome

- Incidence = 1:12,000
- **C**oloboma = defect of the eye (iris, choroid, retina, disc or optic nerve)
- **H**eart defects = conotruncal and arch abnormalities
- **A**tresia of the choanae = airway obstruction, no patency of airway passage to nasopharynx
- **R**etardation of growth and/or development
- **G**enitourinary / **G**astrointestinal = GERD, omphalocele, anal atresia or stenosis
- **E**ar anomalies
- Developmental delay, vision and hearing loss
- Upper airway abnormalities in 56% of children

VACTERL Association

- **V**ertebral anomalies - hemi vertebrae, fused or dysplastic vertebrae
- **A**nal atresia, imperforate anus
- **C**ardiac defects - ¾ of these children have congenital heart disease
- **T**racheoesophageal fistula and/or **E**sophageal atresia
- **R**enal anomalies
- **L**imb, radial atresia

Difficult Airway Syndromes

- Pierre Robin syndrome = **micrognathia**, glossoptosis, respiratory distress, +/- cleft palate
- Goldenhar syndrome = unilateral hemifacial microsomia, mandibular retrognathia, absent ear
- Treacher Collins syndrome = mandibular hypoplasia, macrosomia, cleft palate
- Hurler/Hunter syndrome = mucopolysaccharidosis type I/II disorders, coarse facial features, widely-spaced teeth, macroglossia, coarse facies
- Beckwith-Wiedemann syndrome = macroglossia, gigantism, organomegaly. May or may not be a difficult airway.

Congenital Diaphragmatic Hernia (CDH)

- 1:2,000 live births
- Most common type:
    - Foramen of Bochdalek: opening in the posterior lateral (more commonly left side) diaphragm
- Other types:
    - Morgagni anterior portion of diaphragm
    - Hiatus
- Mortality 50%
- Si/Sx: acidosis, hypoxia, respiratory distress, scaphoid abdomen
- Chest X-ray: loops of bowel in chest (left side = most common), mediastinal displacement
    - CXR also useful to rule out pneumothorax
- **Pulmonary hypertension** - determines morbidity and mortality
- Pulmonary hypoplasia
    - Ipsilateral side: 20% of lung remains normal
    - Contralateral side: 60 – 70% of lung remains normal
- Right sided lesions associated with increased M&M
- Treatment goals:
    - "Permissive hypercapnia"
        - Low tidal volumes
    - Muscular paralysis to reduce VO_2, decrease work of breathing
    - Avoid bag-mask ventilation
        - Risk: insufflations of stomach which decreases ability to ventilate
    - ECMO: used as last resort
        - Usually determined by severity of pulmonary HTN and degree of hypoxia
- Proceed to surgery when hemodynamically stable
    - Risk: pneumothorax - sudden deterioration in lung compliance or hemodynamic instability

Abdominal Defects

Omphalocele

- 1:5,000 births
- Abdominal defect covered with a membrane
- Umbilicus continuous with sac
- Failure of yolk sac development
- Frequently associated anomalies
    - Prematurity
    - GI anomalies
    - GU anomalies
    - Congenital heart disease
    - Beckwith-Wiedemann syndrome: visceromegaly, hypoglycemia, polycythemia, macroglossia
- Tend to be hemodynamically stable, bowel usually normal

Gastroschisis

- 1:15,000 births
  Abdominal viscera exposed
- Umbilicus lateral to defect
- Failure of omphalomesenteric artery
- Usually an isolated congenital anomaly
- Potential high morbidity, exposed gut = loss of fluids high, abnormal bowel

Omphalocele/Gastroschisis Concerns

- Full Stomach: RSI induction
- Decompress stomach: nasogastric (NG) or orogastric (OG) tube
- Abdominal content closure = may present as abdominal compartment syndrome
    - Increased peak airway pressures
    - Decreased organ perfusion
    - Decreased ability to ventilate
- If defect is large, may require staged closure
- If peak inspiratory pressures increase and unable to ventilate, open the abdomen
- Most of these patients now come to OR after silo (clear plastic or silicone bag) has been placed to cover the defect
    - Initiates abdominal content reduction gradually
    - Reduces heat loss
    - Keeps abdominal contents moist

Duchenne Muscular Dystrophy

- X-linked recessive = mother carrier (**XX**) to son (**XY**)
- Dystrophin = protein present in muscle: striated, cardiac, and smooth
    - DMD dystrophin is absent or non-functional
- Onset: 2 – 6 years old with weakness of pelvic girdle
    - Increased difficulty rising from sitting to standing position
    - Classic sign = pseudohypertrophy of calf muscles
- Cardiac abnormalities: arrhythmias, r/o dilated cardiomyopathy, check ECHO
- GERD common
- Scoliosis usually severe
- Respiratory compromise, presents as restrictive pulmonary disease
- Loss of ambulation by age 10
- **Succinylcholine = ABSOLUTE contraindication**
    - Risk for **lethal hyperkalemia**
    - Duchenne is the reason for the black box warning on succinylcholine
- **Volatile Anesthetics = possible rhabdomyolysis**
    - TIVA recommended
- Duchenne is NOT an known disease risk for malignant hyperthermia

DiGeorge Syndrome

- 1: 3,000 births
- Chromosome 22q deletion
- Also known as velocardiofacial syndrome (VCFS)
- Dysmorphic facial features
    - Small mouth / teeth
    - Down-turned mouth
    - Hypertelorism (wide-set eyes)
- Conotruncal cardiac anomalies
- Thymus: absent or small
    - T-cell abnormalities, immunodeficiency
    - Irradiated blood products required
- Hypoparathyroidism
    - Hypocalcemia
    - Tetany or seizure
- Developmental delays, ADHD, speech delays

Pyloric Stenosis

- 1:800 live births
- Male > female
- Acquired disorder, presents typically 3-8 weeks old
- Concentric hypertrophy radial smooth muscle of pylorus
    - Classically "olive-shaped mass" felt in abdomen
- Diagnosis: ultrasound
- Si/Sx: projectile vomiting (non-bilious)
    - Volume contraction causes **METABOLIC ALKALOSIS**
    - Dehydration: sunken fontanelles, dry mucous membranes, lethargy, tachycardia, decreased urine output, mottled skin = sign of lactic acidosis
- Medical emergency 2° to hypovolemia/metabolic derangements
- Electrolyte abnormalities:
    - **HYPOkalemia**
    - **HYPOchloremia**
    - **Metabolic alkalosis**
    - Paradoxical aciduria
    - Dehydration severity:
        - Mild $\quad$ Cl > 100
        - Moderate $\quad$ Cl = 90-100
        - Severe $\quad$ Cl < 90
- Immediate medical intervention: Fluid resuscitation
    - 20 ml/kg NS bolus
    - Maintenance D5 ½ NS with 20 mEq KCl (potassium chloride)
    - Only add potassium once baby has made urine
- Treatment goals once volume resuscitated:
    - Recheck labs (basic metabolic panel)
    - Surgery: laparoscopic pyloromyotomy
        - Empty Stomach PRIOR to rapid sequence induction
        - RSI, full stomach regardless of NPO duration
        - Rapid sequence induction with succinylcholine or rocuronium, ETT with stylet
- NPO, continue maintenance fluids with glucose
- Respiratory effort may be depressed due to compensatory changes in cerebral spinal fluid
- ***** AVOID OPIOIDS *****

Tracheoesophageal Fistula

- 1:4,000 live births
- 30 – 50% have additional anomalies, i.e. VACTERL association, please check ECHO report
- Si/Sx: coughing, choking, cyanosis with feeds, increased oral secretions, abdomen tympanic (air), inability to pass NG/OG tube
- Concerns: aspiration, pulmonary complications, hypoxemia
- Several different types classified by letters
    - Type "C" = 80 – 85%, esophageal atresia with distal tracheoesophageal fistula
    - Type H = can be confused with tracheoesophageal cleft
- Goals:
    - Decrease oral secretions with continuous suction, oral/esophageal tube
    - Occlude fistula with Fogarty catheter
    - Consider venting stomach with G-tube
    - Maintain spontaneous ventilation
    - Avoid increased PIP to diminish likelihood of insufflating stomach via fistula
    - Placement of ETT - usually distal to fistula is ideal
- These patients return frequently post-op for esophageal dilation procedures
- Concern: incomplete repair or new fistula formation
- Many of these patients have chronic lung disease (2° to chronic aspiration)

Neuroblastoma

- Tumor of postganglionic adrenergic cell
- Arises anywhere along sympathetic ganglion chain
    - Most frequently arises from adrenal glands
    - Posterior mediastinal mass
- 75% secrete catecholamines
    - HTN secondary to catecholamines
- Compression of renal circulation from mass effect
- Si/Sx: flushing, diaphoresis, diarrhea, HTN, abdominal mass
- Von Recklinghausen disease (neurofibromatosis type 1): neuroblastoma, pheochromocytoma

Wilms Tumor

- Wilms tumor = **nephro**blastoma
- Incidence 1:13,000
- Most common abdominal tumor (renal tumor)
- 6 months – 5 years old
- Retroperitoneal/large abdominal mass
- Lung most common site of metastasis
- Treatment: Doxorubicin (Adriamycin) - cardiotoxic if dose >300 mg/m^2
- Invasion of IVC: 4 – 10% cases
- Right atrium thrombus: <1% cases
- HTN 60% cases secondary to renin secretion, ACE inhibitors preferred
- Secondary hyperaldosteronism and hypokalemia may be present

Down Syndrome

- Chromosome #21, trisomy
- Intellectual and developmental delays
- Common Features: "flattened facies", protruding tongue (relative macroglossia), slanting eyes, space between 1st and 2nd toe, single palmar crease
- Frequent congenital anomalies:
    - Cardiac: VSD, AV canal
    - GI: Biliary atresia, Hirschsprung disease (blockage of large intestine)
    - Musculoskeletal: C1 – C2 subluxation (neck X-rays in school age children for sports participation concerns), hypotonia, head flexion is greater concern than extension
    - Heme/Onc: anemia, increased risk leukemia (most common: AMKL - acute megakaryoblastic leukemia)
    - Endocrine: hypothyroidism
    - ENT: OSA extremely common, frequent ear infections
- Anesthesia concerns: obstructive sleep apnea!!! opioid-sensitive, bradycardia with mask induction common
- Congenital heart disease common, check ECHO

ECMO Criteria

- Pre-ductal (i.e. measure at right hand) O_2 saturation <85%,
- Oxygenation Index (OI) >40
    - OI = (FiO_2 × Mean Airway Pressure)/PaO_2
    - PIP >28
- Persistent metabolic acidosis
- Hypotension refractory to pressor support
- Veno-arterial (VA) = most commonly used for cardiac disease (pump failure), and hemodynamic instability
- Veno-venous (VV) = most commonly used for respiratory failure, i.e. RSV

TORCH Syndrome

- Perinatal infections causing severe fetal anomalies
- **T**oxoplasmosis - prematurity, IUGR, hepatosplenomegaly, myocarditis
- **O**ther agents
- **R**ubella - microcephaly, deafness, chorioretinitis, hepatosplenomegaly, thrombocytopenia
- **C**MV - clinically similar to Rubella
- **H**erpes - visceral organ involvement, DIC, encephalitis

Scoliosis

- Scoliosis = lateral deviation of spine >10°
- Cobb angle used to measure magnitude of curve, antero-posterior (AP) X-ray
    - 45° usually required for surgical intervention
- Classification: idiopathic vs non-idiopathic
    - Idiopathic = otherwise completely healthy patient
    - Non-idiopathic (Duchenne, cerebral palsy, spinal muscle atrophy)
- Pulmonary impairment pre-operative and post-op
    - Pre-op spirometry testing will show a RESTRICTIVE LUNG DEFECT
        - FVC most important predictor of post op impairment
        - Degree of impairment directly related to degree of thoracic curve
        - Long term pulmonary consequences of uncorrected spine - hypoxemia, recurrent infections, pulmonary hypertension
    - Post-op complications 5X more likely in non-idiopathic
        - Consider post-op ventilation if FVC <30%
        - FVC and FEV1 decreased 40 – 50% of baseline POD #1, return to baseline 1 – 2 mos postoperatively
- SSEP/ MEP monitoring used for spinal cord function surveillance
    - Considered significant and intervention required when:
        - Increased latency >10%
        - Decreased amplitude >50%
    - Increased risk in watershed area T4 – T9, region of poorest blood supply
    - Motor signals are most vulnerable
    - TIVA recommended, multiple anesthetics have direct effect on SSEP/ MEP
    - Factors that increase possibility of spinal cord injury:
        - Pedicle screws
        - Hypoperfusion
        - Direct contusion
        - Mechanical-distraction
- Surgical EBL
    - Idiopathic scoliosis: 750 – 1,500 ml
    - Non-idiopathic scoliosis: 2,500 – 4,000 ml
- Pain management: consider multi-modal technique: intrathecal morphine, gabapentin, Tylenol, patient-controlled analgesia (PCA)

Chapter 6: Pediatric Advanced Life Support

- ❖ Neonatal Resuscitation
- ❖ Pediatric CPR
- ❖ Bradycardia
- ❖ Epinephrine Facts
- ❖ Pediatric Perioperative Cardiac Arrest

Neonatal Resuscitation

Algorithm for resuscitation

- **Term gestation? Breathing or crying? Good tone?**
    - Yes – Stay with mother → Provide routine care
    - No – Warm, clear airway, dry, stimulate (continue below)
- **HR below 100, gasping, or apnea?**
    - No – Labored breathing or persistent cyanosis?
        - No → Provide routine care
        - Yes → Clear airway, SpO$_2$ monitoring*, consider CPAP
          → Post-resuscitation care
    - Yes → Positive pressure ventilation, SpO$_2$ monitoring
- **HR below 100?**
    - No → Post-resuscitation care
    - Yes → Take ventilation corrective steps
- **HR below 60?**
    - No → Go back to "HR below 100" bullet point
    - Yes → Consider intubation, Chest compressions, Coordinate with PPV
- **HR still below 60?**
    - Yes → Give IV epinephrine until above
    - Intubate if not getting chest rise
    - Consider hypovolemia or pneumothorax

> *** Targeted Pre-ductal SpO$_2$ after birth**
> - 1 min: 60 – 65%
> - 2 min: 65 – 70%
> - 3 min: 70 – 75%
> - 4 min: 75 – 80%
> - 5 min: 80 – 85%
> - 10 min: 85 – 90%

Adapted from 2010 American Heart Association

Pediatric CPR

Asystole, PEA

- Call for help
- Give 100% oxygen. Turn off all anesthetic gases. Place patient on backboard.
- Start chest compressions **(100 chest compressions/min + 8 breaths/min)**
    - Maintain good hand position
    - Maximize $ETCO_2$ >10 mm Hg with force/ depth of compressions
    - Allow full recoil between compressions.
    - Switch with another provider every 2 minutes, if possible.
    - Use sudden increase in $ETCO_2$ for return on spontaneous circulation (ROSC)
    - Do not stop compressions for pulse check
- **Epinephrine 10 mcg/kg IV q 3 – 5 min**
- Check pulse & rhythm (q 2 min during compressor switch)
- Call for ECMO (if available) if no return of spontaneous circulation after 6 min of CPR

V-Fib/V-tach

- Call for help and defibrillator
- Give 100% oxygen. Turn off all anesthetic gases. Place patient on backboard.
- Start chest compressions **(100 chest compressions/min + 8 breaths/min)**
    - Maintain good hand position
    - Maximize $ETCO_2$ >10 mm Hg with force/depth of compressions
    - Allow full recoil between compressions – lift hands off chest
- **Shock 2 – 4 joules/kg**
- Resume chest compressions x 2 min
- **Epinephrine 10 mcg/kg IV q 3-5 min**
- Check pulse & rhythm (q 2 min during compressor switch)
- If shockable rhythm continues:
    - **Shock 4 joules/kg**
    - Resume chest compressions x 2 min
    - Epinephrine 10 mcg/kg IV
    - Check pulse & rhythm (q 2 min during compressor switch)
    - Shock 4 – 10 joules/kg, continue chest compressions, and epinephrine 10 mcg/kg IV every 3 – 5min
    - Amiodarone 5 mg/kg bolus IV; may repeat x 2
- Call for ECMO (if available) after 6 min of CPR

Adapted from 2010 American Heart Association.

Bradycardia

Age	HR
<30 d	<100
>30 d – <1 yr	<80
>1 yr	<60

- Call for help and transcutaneous pacer
- **Hypoxia is common cause of bradycardia in pediatric population**
    - Ensure patient is not hypoxic, give 100% oxygen
- Stop surgical stimulation. If laparoscopy, desufflate
- Turn off anesthetic gases
- Consider
    - Epinephrine 2 – 10 mcg/kg IV
    - Chest compression if pulseless or pulse <60 beats/min
- Assess for drug-induced causes
- Beta-blocker overdose: glucagon 0.05 mg/kg IV, then 0.07 mg/kg/h IV infusion
    - Calcium channel blocker overdose: calcium chloride 10 – 20 mg/kg IV or calcium gluconate 50 mg/kg, then glucagon if calcium ineffective
- Note: atropine is no longer considered drug of choice for bradycardia that is due to hypoxia

Adapted from 2010 American Heart Association.

Epinephrine Facts

- Alpha 1, alpha 2, beta 1, and beta 2 agonist
    - Beta 1: myocardium effects, increased blood pressure, cardiac output, oxygen demand
    - Alpha 1: decreased splanchnic blood flow, **increased coronary perfusion** (vasoconstriction)
    - Beta 2: relaxes bronchial smooth muscle
    - Myocardium = beta receptors: 70% beta 1
- Coronary perfusion pressure = diastolic pressure – LVEDP (or wedge pressure)
- Code doses:
    - 0.01 mg/kg (0.1 ml/kg 1:10,000) IV/IO
    - 0.1 mg/kg (0.1 ml/kg 1:1000) ETT
    - Maximum dose 1 mg IV/ IO; 2.5 mg ETT
- ADRS
    - May cause ventricular ectopy, tachyarrhythmias, vasoconstriction, and hypertension
    - Caution: Do not administer catecholamines and sodium bicarbonate simultaneously through an IV catheter or tubing, alkaline solutions such as the bicarbonate inactivate the catecholamines

Pediatric Perioperative Cardiac Arrest

- Pediatric Perioperative Cardiac Arrest (POCA) Registry: data collection regarding cardiac arrest and deaths during administration or recovery from anesthesia in United States
- Multicenter participation, voluntary
- Initial findings 1994 – 1997, Morray *et al.*, Anesthesiology, July 2000
- Updated findings 1998 – 2004
    - 397 reported events, 49% related to anesthesia
    - Causes of events
        - Cardiovascular - 41%
        - Respiratory - 27%
        - Medication - 18%
        - Equipment - 5%
    - Phase of anesthetic
        - Maintenance - 58%
        - Pre-induction/induction - 24%
        - Emergence - 19%
- Cardiovascular Events
    - Hypovolemia from blood loss #1 etiology
    - Electrolyte imbalance
        - Hyperkalemia from transfusion of stored blood
- Respiratory Events
    - Laryngospasm #1 etiology

Bhananker MD et al. Anesthesia-Related Cardiac Arrest in Children: Update from the Pediatric Perioperative Cardiac Arrest Registry, International Anesthesia Research Society, Vol 105, No.2, 2007, P344-350.

Chapter 7: Malignant Hyperthermia

- ❖ Associated Diseases
- ❖ Inheritance Pattern
- ❖ Pharmacology
- ❖ MH Signs/Symptoms
- ❖ Differential Diagnosis
- ❖ Definitive Diagnosis
- ❖ Treatment/Interventions
- ❖ Dantrolene

Associated Diseases

- Definitive relationship with these skeletal muscle myopathies:
    - **Central core disease**
    - **Multiminicore disease**
    - **King-Denborough syndrome**
- Other myopathies, such as Duchenne and Becker are not directly associated with MH

Inheritance Pattern

- Autosomal dominant with variable penetrance
- Considered a "pharmacogenetic" disease
- Incidence: child 1:15,000 vs adult 1 : 50,000
- Ryanodine receptor (RyR_1): regulates intracellular Ca^{2+} fluxes
- Chromosome #19, with others likely associated
- Susceptible patients can have repeated exposures prior to MH reaction

Pharmacology

- The following agents trigger MH
    - Succinylcholine
    - All volatile anesthetics
    - Heat/exercise/stress
- All other medications given for anesthesia are safe
- N_2O is NOT considered a volatile agent and is safe to use
- **Hypermetabolic syndrome**, trigger agents cause sustained muscle contraction
    - "Charlie horse" contraction throughout body
    - Increased VO_2
    - Increased CO_2
    - Increased extracellular K^+

MH Signs/Symptoms

- Heart involvement – unexplained arrhythmias, ST, VT, VF
- Tachypnea
- Mixed metabolic/respiratory acidosis
- Base excess <−8 or pH <7.25
- **ETCO$_2$ >55 mmHg or PaCO$_2$ >60 mmHg**
- Muscle rigidity – generalized rigidity including severe masseter muscle rigidity
- Muscle breakdown – rhabdomyolysis
    - CK >20,000/L units
    - Cola- colored urine, myoglobinuria
    - K$^+$ >6 mEq/L
- Temperature increase – rapidly increasing temperature, (T >38.8 °C)
- Hallmark of MH is a complete inability to reduce CO$_2$, despite ventilation changes

Differential Diagnosis

- Heat stroke
- Propofol infusion syndrome
- Neuroleptic malignant syndrome
- Serotonin syndrome

Definitive Diagnosis

- Caffeine halothane contracture test
    - Will capture all at risk, gold standard test for diagnosis
    - Must be performed at testing center, 4 centers in US
    - Discouraged in pre-pubescent children
- Genetics - blood sample
    - Will only capture 30% of those at risk
    - Can send blood sample via mail
    - Two centers in United States
- Rx: ryanodine receptor gene test for MH susceptibility
- Malignant Hyperthermia Association of United States = MHAUS
    - 24-hour MH hotline
    - 1-800-644-9737

Treatment/Interventions

- CALL FOR HELP
- Get malignant hyperthermia (MH) kit/cart
- Stop procedure if possible
- Stop volatile anesthetic, give 100% O_2
- Transition to non-triggering anesthetic (Propofol, opioids)
- Request chilled IV saline
- **Hyperventilate** patient to reduce CO_2: 2 – 4 times patient's minute ventilation
- **Change anesthesia circuit**
- **Dantrolene 2.5 mg/kg IV every 5 min** until symptoms resolve
    - Assign dedicated person to mix dantrolene (20 mg/vial) in 60 ml sterile water
- **Bicarbonate 1 – 2 mEq/kg IV** for suspected metabolic acidosis; maintain pH >7.2
- **Cool patient** if temperature >38.5 °C
    - Nasogastric lavage with cold water
    - Apply ice externally
    - Infuse cold saline intravenously
    - ** Stop cooling if temperature <38 °C
- Hyperkalemia treatment
    - Calcium gluconate (30 mg/kg IV) or calcium chloride (10 mg/kg IV)
    - Sodium bicarbonate (1 – 2 mEq/kg IV)
    - Regular insulin 10 Units IV with 1 – 2 amps D50% (0.1 units insulin/kg and 1 ml/kg D50%)
- Dysrhythmia treatment
    - Standard anti-arrhythmic—DO NOT use calcium channel blocker
- Send labs:
    - ABG or VBG, electrolytes, serum CPK, serum/urine myoglobin, coagulation
- Place Foley catheter to monitor urine output
- Call ICU to arrange disposition.
- Once patient is stabilized, and critical event over, contact MHAUS hotline
    - 1-800-644-9737

Dantrolene

- Muscle relaxant
- Decreases release of Ca^{2+} from sarcoplasmic reticulum
- Patient will be weak with treatment, and post-op vent support should be considered necessary
- Recrudescence= reoccurrence
    - 20% chance of recrudescence
    - Predictors of increased risk:
        - Muscular body type
        - Delayed reaction = increased duration from exposure to MH reaction
- Dantrolene dose
    - Initial dose: 2.5 mg/kg IV up to 10 mg/kg
    - Post-op: 1 ml/kg every 6 hours for 24 – 48 hours as necessary
- Thrombophlebitis possible
- Ryanodex = new formulation
    - 1 vial = 250 mg
    - Mix with 5 ml water only
    - Initial dose: 2.5 mg/kg IV

Chapter 8: Regional Anesthesia/Pain

- ❖ Local Anesthetics: Overview
- ❖ Local Anesthetics: Differences in Pediatrics
- ❖ Local Anesthetics: Toxic Doses
- ❖ Epinephrine
- ❖ EMLA
- ❖ Methemoglobinemia
- ❖ Dibucaine Number
- ❖ Pediatric Neuraxial Anesthesia
- ❖ Transversus Abdominis Plane (TAP) Block
- ❖ Complex Regional Pain Syndromes

Local Anesthetics: Overview

- Onset = pKa (exception: chloroprocaine, rapid onset despite higher pKa = 9)
- Duration of action = protein binding
- Potency = lipid solubility
- Plasma protein binding determines CV risks, free unbound protein produces toxicity
- Positive test dose with local anesthetic (typically 1% lido + 1:200,000 epinephrine)
    - Increased T wave amplitude >25 %, most reliable, happens within 30 sec
    - Increased HR >10 beats per minute
    - Increased SBP >15 mmHg

Local Anesthetics: Differences in Pediatrics

- Greater cardiac output to vessel rich groups → greater uptake of drug
    - Higher risk for toxicity
    - Shorter duration of action
- Decreased plasma proteins prior to age 3 – 6 months
    - Higher toxicity risk due to increased free fraction of drug
- Toxicity primarily two systems: CNS and CV
    - CNS: seizure
        - Likely cannot assess 1st Si/Sx of neurotoxicity in infant
        - Likely cannot assess when blocks performed under GA
    - CV: arrhythmias/ cardiovascular collapse
        - Ventricular tachycardia/arrest, bradycardia, conduction blocks, widening QRS, torsades, new onset PVCs
- Toxicity treatment with lipid emulsion = 20% intralipid
    - Acts as a "drug sink" pulling drug from myocardial conduction pathway
    - Propofol is 10% intralipid but causes SVR drop and is no substitute
    - Dose 1.5 ml/kg and 0.25 ml/kg/min with up to 2 repeat boluses 3 minutes apart until return of spontaneous circulation (ROSC)
    - Risks from lipid emulsion: thrombophlebitis, inflammatory response, anaphylaxis, increased risk acute pancreatitis

Local Anesthetics: Toxic Doses

Bupivacaine	With epinephrine: 2.5 mg/kg
	Infants <6 mo: 2 mg/kg)
Chloroprocaine	With epinephrine: 11 – 14 mg/kg
Lidocaine	With epinephrine: 5 – 7 mg/kg
Mepivacaine	7 mg/kg
Ropivacaine	5 mg/kg

Epinephrine

- Used in regional blocks, as well as neuraxial test doses
- Continuous infusion has been described as detrimental in "at risk populations" by Pediatric Regional Anesthesia Network (PRAN)
- Epi causes vasoconstriction which delays uptake, and prolongs block
- Used in test dose with lidocaine to determine if intravascular
- 1:200,000 common concentration of epinephrine added to local anesthetics for regional block procedures
- Concentration = dose/ volume

$$1 \text{ gm} : 200,000 \text{ ml}$$
$$1000 \text{ mg} : 200,000 \text{ ml}$$
$$1000 \text{ mcg} : 200 \text{ ml}$$
$$10 \text{ mcg} : 2 \text{ ml}$$
$$\mathbf{5 \text{ mcg} : 1 \text{ ml}}$$

EMLA Cream

- Mixture of local anesthetics = lidocaine + prilocaine
- Topical agent, 45 – 60 min onset
- Used for IV punctures, placement of Huber needles into implanted ports
- ADRs: methemoglobinemia, skin blanching
- Contraindicated:
    - Infants <1 mos old
    - Infants <1 yr old receiving methemoglobin-inducing agents

Methemoglobinemia

- Hemoglobin - Fe^{2+} ions(ferrous) becomes reduced to Fe^{3+} (ferric) which cannot bind O_2
- Hb-O_2 dissociation curve is shifted to the **left**
- Clinical presentation
    - Cyanotic features
    - "Chocolate" brown-colored blood
- Normal PaO_2
- **SpO_2 at 85%**, saturation does not increase with supplemental oxygen
- Methemoglobin-inducing agents: nitrate-containing drugs including benzocaine, prilocaine, dapsone, nitric oxide, and lidocaine, iNO
- Tx: methylene blue + 100% O_2

Dibucaine Number

- Test for abnormal pseudocholinesterase activity
- Dibucaine is an **amide** local anesthetic
- Pseudocholinesterase enzyme responsible for metabolism of succinylcholine
- **Dibucaine # = % inhibition of pseudocholinesterase enzyme**
    - 80% inhibition = homozygous normal response
    - 60% inhibition = heterozygous normal response
    - 20% inhibition = homozygous atypical = PROFOUND prolonged block from succinylcholine

Pediatric Neuraxial Anesthesia

Spinal
- Spinal anatomy
    - Spinal cord ends (conus medullaris)
        - Adult – L1
        - Infant – L3
    - Dural sac ends
        - Adult – S1
        - Infant – S3
- Spinal physiology
    - Total CSF volume increased in infants 4 ml/kg vs 2 ml/kg for adults
    - Hydrostatic pressure decreased in infants, 30 – 40 cm H_2O lower
    - Infants require higher ml/kg dose of local anesthetic, 2° to increased volume of distribution
    - Narcotic effect is 10-fold greater in spinal (intrathecal) than epidural space

Caudal

- Caudal block is an epidural block performed at the level of the sacrum
- Caudal anatomy
    - Sacrum, PSIS
    - Sacral cornu = bony landmark
        - Formed by incomplete fusion of sacral vertebral arch
    - Needle pierces the sacrococcygeal ligament
        - Ligament continuously developing/ossifying until ceases at age 8 yo
    - Hiatus typically between cornu, but may be above or below due to several very common anatomical variants
    - Sacral dimple raises index of suspicion for undiagnosed tether, or other neuraxial aberrancy
        - Dimples occur in 3 – 10% of children but neuraxial aberrancy is rare
- Caudal physiology
    - Caudal has been shown to increase PVR indices - do not use in severe pulm HTN
    - Volume determines dermatome
        - Sacral 0.5 ml/kg
        - Lower thorax 1 ml/kg
        - Mid thorax 1.25 ml/kg
    - Complications: epidural abscess, epidural hematoma, intra-vascular injection, spinal injection, LAST (Local Anesthetic Systemic Toxicity)
    - Narcotic effect : spinal 10X > epidural; epidural 10X > intravenous

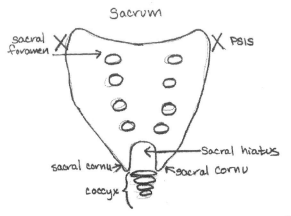

Transversus Abdominis Plane (TAP) Block

- Dermatomes T7 – L1
- Large volume-based block
    - Typically 0.2 ml/kg per side (be aware of maximum doses)
- Anatomical approach
    - Lumbar triangle of Petit: latissimus dorsi, external oblique, and iliac crest
    - Two muscle pops:
        - Penetration of external oblique fascia
        - Entry into plane between internal oblique and transversus abdominis muscles
    - Challenging to assess in obese
- Ultrasound approach
    - Axial probe placement lateral to umbilicus
    - Slide lateral until three muscle groups visualized
    - Superficial to deep: external/internal/transversus abdominis
- Needle tip between internal oblique and transverse abdominus
- Greater success with more lateral placement of volume (nerves come lateral to medial)
- Does not cover visceral pain, only somatic and incisional pain

Chronic Regional Pain Syndromes

CRPS 1
- Formerly known as reflex sympathetic dystrophy (RSD)
- Si/Sx : allodynia, cyanosis, mottling coldness, atrophy, temperature changes, decreased range of motion
- Diagnosis of CRPS is typically a diagnosis of exclusion
- Triple phase bone scan can show abnormalities and aid in diagnosis
- Categories for clinical diagnosis: Budapest criteria
- Sensory, vasomotor, sudomotor/edema, motor/trophic
- Female > male
- Lower extremity > upper extremity

CRPS 2
- Formerly known as causalgia
    - Injury follows a known nerve distribution, has a known "cause"
- Described by physicians during the American Civil War in soldiers with peripheral nerve injuries from bullets or shrapnel who reported a burning quality to their pain
- Treatment:
    - Sympathetic block,
    - Physical therapy (early desensitization therapy)
    - Transcutaneous electrical nerve stimulation (TENS)
    - Spinal cord stimulation
- Successful sympathetic block = temperature change in targeted limb after block
- Kuntz fibers are sympathetic fibers that do not travel through sympathetic ganglion. These fibers may be missed by regional block.
- CRPS does not always have to be sympathetically mediated.
- Rx: tricyclics, gabapentin, bisphosphonates

Budapest Criteria for CRPS

1. Continuing pain, which is disproportionate to any inciting event
2. Must report at least one symptom in three of the four following categories:
   - Sensory: reports of hyperesthesia and/or allodynia
   - Vasomotor: reports of temperature asymmetry and/or skin color changes and/or skin color asymmetry
   - Sudomotor/edema: reports of edema and/or sweating changes and/or sweating asymmetry
   - Motor/trophic: reports of decreased range of motion and/or motor dysfunction (weakness, tremor, dystonia) and/or trophic changes (hair, nail, skin)
3. Must display at least one sign at time of evaluation in two or more of the following categories:
   - Sensory: evidence of hyperalgesia (to pinprick) and/or allodynia (to light touch and/or deep somatic pressure and/or joint movement)
   - Vasomotor: evidence of temperature asymmetry and/or skin color changes and/or asymmetry
   - Sudomotor/edema: evidence of edema and/or sweating changes and/or sweating asymmetry
   - Motor/trophic: evidence of decreased range of motion and/or motor dysfunction (weakness, tremor, dystonia) and/or trophic changes (hair, nail, skin)
4. There is no other diagnosis that better explains the signs and symptoms

Chapter 9: Neurosurgery Topics

- ❖ Neurological Development
- ❖ Meningomyelocele
- ❖ Cerebral Palsy
- ❖ Arnold Chiari Malformation
- ❖ Hydrocephalus
- ❖ AV Malformation
- ❖ Moyamoya
- ❖ Cranial Tumors
- ❖ Craniosynostosis
- ❖ Venous Air Embolism
- ❖ Traumatic Brain Injury
- ❖ Diuretics
- ❖ Diabetes Insipidus vs SIADH

Neurological Development

- Brain growth
    - 15 – 20 weeks: neuronal cell multiplication
    - 25 weeks – 2yrs: glial cell multiplication
    - Up to 3 years: myelination continues
- Fontanelles
    - Openings in skull, bones not fused at birth
    - Anterior = formed by 2 frontal bones (closes at 9 – 18 months)
    - Posterior = junction of 2 parietal bones (closes at 4 months)
- Sutures
    - Metopic, coronal, sagittal, lambdoid
- Cerebral blood flow
    - Adult: 55 ml/100g brain tissue/min (15% cardiac output)
    - Child: 100 ml/100g brain tissue/min (25% cardiac output)
    - Neonate: 40 ml/100g brain tissue/min
- $CMRO_2$ Adult 3.5 – 4.5 ml O_2/100g/min, increased in child
- Pediatrics decreased intracranial compliance, 2° to increased brain H_2O content
- Intracranial pressures – normal values
    - Adult: ICP < 15mmHg
    - Child: ICP 3 – 7 mmHg
    - Neonate: ICP 1.5 – 6 mmHg
- Si/Sx of increased intracranial pressure
    - **Cushing reflex= HTN + bradycardia**
    - N/V, altered mental status, lethargy
    - Eyes: "setting sun" sign, papilledema, pupillary dilation or unequal pupils
    - These Si/Sx may be absent in young children
    - Check pupils pre-op, pupils don't lie (unless atropine was given)

Meningomyelocele

- 1:1000 live births
- Neural tube defect = sac-like herniation of neural tissue + meninges
- Most common in lumbosacral region 75%
- Most present with paralysis below level of defect, urinary/bowel incontinence
- Usually come to operating room as newborn for defect repair, day 1 – 2 of life
- Common associations: Arnold Chiari II, tethered cord, short trachea, hydrocephalus
- Concerns: cranial nerve palsies, hypothermia (large surface area exposed), blood loss
- Monitoring: +/- SSEP
- Positioning: prone
- High-risk for latex allergy
- No abnormal response to succinylcholine, no malignant hyperthermia risks

Cerebral Palsy

- Movement disorder
- Three categories: spastic (70%), dyskinetic, ataxic
- Motor impairment with or without cognitive impairment
- Contractures, hypotonic
- GERD, chronic aspiration
- Seizures
- Decreased MAC by 20%, less volatile anesthetic needed
- Increased sensitivity to NMBs, **PROFOUND** sensitivity to narcotics
- No extra risk of hyperkalemia when given succinylcholine

Arnold Chiari Malformation

- Type I: Cerebellar vermis and medulla oblongata herniate through foramen magnum
- Type II: Additionally associated with meningomyelocele
    - May present in infancy with diminished gag reflexes or vocal cord paralysis
- Aqueduct stenosis, hydrocephalus
- Precautions: extreme head flexion may cause brainstem compression

Hydrocephalus

- Increased ventricles secondary to cerebral spinal fluid
- Increased ICP si/sx common in older children
- Aqueductal stenosis most common cause
- Communicating = obstruction distal to ventricles
- Non-communicating = obstruction within ventricles
- Tx: ventriculoperitoneal (VP) vs ventriculoatrial (VA) shunt

AV Malformation

- Abnormal communication between arterial and venous systems
- **Intracranial hemorrhage most common presentation**
- May present as CHF in infancy = high flow output failure, may require inotrope/pressor support
- Most go undetected until 4th/5th decade of life
- Common in peds: posterior cerebral artery and great cerebral vein (vein of Galen)
- Tx: embolization vs surgical excision

Moyamoya

- Occlusion of intracranial vessels
    - Internal carotid/circle of Willis
- Associated with: Down syndrome and Neurofibromatosis type I, Sickle cell, and Japanese ancestry
- "Puff of smoke" angiographic appearance, TIAs common
- Very sensitive to CO_2, avoid decreased CO_2 = vasoconstriction
- Precautions
    - **Normocarbia critical**
    - Increased risks stroke during anesthesia
    - Maintain BP w/in 20% baseline
    - Ketamine not recommended

Cranial Tumors

- 2nd most common cancer in pediatrics, #1 is leukemia
- Supratentorial 15 - 20%:
    - Astrocytoma, glioblastomas, oligodendroglioma, meningioma
    - Visual disturbances + endocrine
    - Si/Sx: seizure disorder + focal deficits
- Posterior Fossa = 45 – 60%, most common
    - 30% medulloblastoma M>F
    - 30% cerebellar astrocytoma
    - 30% brainstem glioma
    - Si/Sx: usually obstruction of 4th ventricle, CN palsies, ataxia, headache

Craniosynostosis

- Premature fusion of cranial sutures
    - Cosmetic deformity
    - Possible increased ICP
- Sagittal suture most common
- Craniofacial syndromes common (Apert, Crouzon) or idiopathic
- Usually repaired in infancy, under 1 year old
    - May require staged repair
- Bleeding major concern, multiple intravenous access and arterial line standard
- Venous air embolism possible
- Dislodgement of endotracheal tube is a concern, commonly sutured in place
- Possible difficult airway in craniofacial syndrome

Venous Air Embolism

- Gradient between atmospheric pressure and venous pressure
- Operative site higher than heart
    - Crani-posterior
    - Craniosynostosis repair
    - Sitting Crani
    - Laparoscopic procedure
    - Port removal/ placement
    - Spine surgery
    - C-Section
- Venous sinuses (head) have dural attachments that impede ability to collapse
- Monitoring
    - Precordial doppler = most sensitive
    - ECHO = most specific
    - ETN_2 = increased
    - $ETCO_2$ = decreased, dead space increased dramatically
    - Increased right atrial pressure
    - Hypotension, hypoxemia
- Tx: notify surgeon, flood surgical field with saline, position head lower than heart
    - Trendelenburg + left lateral position= traps air in apex of right ventricle, thus preventing obstruction of RV outflow tract, or paradoxical embolus
    - Central venous catheter can be used to aspirate/remove air
    - PALS/ ACLS algorithm

Traumatic Brain Injury

- Most common cause of childhood death and disability
    - Ages at greatest risk: 0 – 4 years old, 15 – 19 years old
- Leading cause of TBI in 0 – 4 years old: falls
- Abusive head trauma/shaken baby syndrome: subdural hematoma, cerebral edema, increased intracranial pressure, neurological deficits
- Depressed skull fracture complications: meningitis, CSF leak, cranial nerve damage
- Epidural hematoma: middle meningeal artery
    - May have lucid period

Centers for Disease Control and Prevention. 2004 Report to Congress. Traumatic Brain Injury in the United States: Emergency Department Visits Hospitalizations, and Deaths.

Diuretics

- Commonly used to decrease ICP
- Hypertonic 3% saline = increases serum osmolality
- Mannitol = osmotic diuretic, onset 10 – 15 min
    - Increases serum osmolality, decreased brain tissue volume 2° decreased water content
    - Initially hypotension 2° vasodilation
    - ADRs: transient increased intravascular volume may lead to pulmonary edema
- Lasix = loop diuretic
    - Decreased brain edema 2° to systemic diuresis
    - ADRs: hypokalemia, metabolic alkalosis, hearing loss

Diabetes Insipidus vs SIADH

Diabetes Insipidus

- May occur post-op crani, trauma
    - 4 cc/kg/hr urine for >1 hr
    - Na^+ 145 mEq/L, **hypernatremia**
    - 300 mOsm serum osmolality
    - <300 mOsm urine osmolality
- Low CVP
- Tx: vasopressin

SIADH

- Syndrome of inappropriate antidiuretic hormone secretion
- Significant number of causes
- Hypervolemia, free H_2O overload
- Decreased urine output
- >280 mOsm serum osmolality, **hyponatremia**
- Urine Na^+ <30 mEq/L
- Tx: 3% saline for Na^+ < 125 mEq/L, Lasix
    - Be aware of rapid correction of Na^+, may develop central pontine myelinolysis
    - Recommendation: should not exceed Na^+ increase of 0.5 mEq/L per hour or 8 – 10 mEq/L/24 hours

Chapter 10: Ear/Nose/Throat Topics

- ❖ Foreign Body in Airway
- ❖ Bleeding Tonsil
- ❖ Tonsillectomy and Adenoidectomy
- ❖ Croup vs Epiglottitis
- ❖ Post-Intubation Croup
- ❖ Obstructive Sleep Apnea
- ❖ Laryngospasm

Foreign Body in Airway

- Airway foreign body may be life-threatening, considered an urgent/emergent case
- Concerns: Complete airway obstruction from foreign object
- Immediate OR if
    - Patient unstable
    - + Respiratory distress, + wheeze, + tachypnea, cyanosis
    - Unable to maintain oxygen saturations
- Blood gas and IVs are usually not immediate concerns
    - Both can upset the child and cause severe dynamic collapse of the airway
- If patient stable, obtain CXR
    - X-rays may be helpful to identify and localize foreign object
    - Food particles may not be radiopaque on CXR
    - +/- Air trapping, +/- tracheal deviation away from affected side
- Peanuts = may have local inflammatory response
    - Unroasted/raw peanut has high oil content compared with roasted peanut
        - Oils evoke inflammatory response that can be severe
- GOALS: Spontaneous respiration + deep level anesthesia
    - Keep child spontaneously breathing for as long as possible
    - Inhalation mask induction ideal, with ENT surgeon present
    - When patient relaxed, you can place IV
- Deepen anesthesia with: dexmedetomidine (Precedex), ketamine, propofol, volatile anesthetic
    - Coughing or patient movement during removal of object can be life threatening, **preventing object from occluding airway is critical**
    - If object completely occludes airway (no ventilation possible), move object down into right or left mainstem—with rigid bronchoscope—to allow ventilation of at least a single lung
- Always have surgeon present when emergent airway is assessed

Bleeding Tonsil

- Emergency
- Full-stomach (blood)
- Review chart from tonsillectomy and adenoidectomy procedure
- Check hemoglobin/ hematocrit, type and cross if necessary
- Rapid sequence induction with cricoid pressure, ETT with stylet
- Prepare two suction canisters
- Most commonly (75%) present within 6 hours post-op
- 2nd most common presentation: post-op day #7 when eschar falls off

Tonsillectomy and Adenoidectomy

- 2nd most common pediatric ambulatory surgery in US, #1 is bilateral myringotomy (BMT)
- Indications:
    - Recurrent infection
    - Sleep disordered breathing: **polysomnography (PSG) = gold standard diagnosis**
    - PSG considered abnormal if O_2 Sat < 92% or ** AHI >1
    - **ASA guideline considers obstructive sleep apnea severe if AHI >10**
- Strong recommendations for:
    - Single intra-op dose IV dexamethasone
    - Strong recommendation AGAINST perioperative antibiotic
- Pain treatment recommendations
    - Tylenol
    - NSAIDs are OK, however ketorolac not recommended!
        - Post-op bleeding with ketorolac 4.4 – 18%
    - Codeine should be avoided
    - Intra-op local anesthetic injection in tonsillar fossa
- Post-Op complications
    - Mortality rates 1 in 16,000 – 1 in 35,000
    - Bleeding
        - Primary = w/in 24 hrs: 0.2 – 2.2%
        - Secondary = >24 hrs: 0.1 – 3%
        - Approximately 1/3 of deaths are attributed to bleeding
    - Airway obstruction, consider long acting narcotics carefully
- Complications more likely: craniofacial disorders, Down syndrome, cerebral palsy, heart defect, bleeding diathesis, patient <3 years old, proven OSA, obesity
- Recommended T&A be done as in-patient procedure for the following patients:
    - Cardiac abnormality, obstructive sleep apnea, neuromuscular disorder, obesity, failure to thrive, recent upper respiratory infections, craniofacial disorder, prematurity
- Overnight hospitalization recommended for:
    - Obese patients
    - Children <3 year old
    - Apnea-hypopnea index (AHI) > 10

Baugh, Reginald et al. 2011. Clinical Practice Guideline: Tonsillectomy in Children. Otolaryngology-Head and Neck Surgery 144(1), S 1-30.

Croup vs Epiglottitis

	CROUP	EPIGLOTTITIS
Location	Subglottic	Supraglottic
Age	Less than 3 y	3 – 6 y
Cause	Viral	Bacterial (Group A Strep*)
Fever	Low grade	High
Drooling	None	Copious
Cough	Present	Absent
X-ray	"Steeple sign"	"Thumb print"
Treatment	O_2 plus humidity	Secure airway, inhalation induction, IV Antibiotics

*H. influenzae unlikely (vaccine available), new etiologies have surfaced

Post-Intubation Croup

- 0.1 – 1% occurrence
- Increased risk occurs:
    - No endotracheal tube air leak >25 cm H_2O
    - Resistance at time of insertion of ETT
    - Changes in patient positioning s/p intubation
    - Repeated and/or traumatic attempts at intubation
    - Coughing on ETT
    - Age 1 – 3 year(s) old
    - Surgery >1 hour
- Tx: humidified mist, nebulized racemic epinephrine, dexamethasone (Decadron)
    - Racemic epinephrine = decrease subglottic mucosal edema
    - Half-life is 0.5 – 2 h
    - Caution: rebound effect once half-life time is up

Obstructive Sleep Apnea

- Apnea = complete cessation of breathing >10 sec
- Hypopnea = 30% reduction in air flow >10 sec
- Apnea-hypopnea index number = # of apneic events/ hour (AHI)
    - 5 – 15 = mild
    - 15 – 30 = moderate
    - >30 severe
- Known predictors of OSA
    - History of prematurity
    - Morbid obesity
    - Nasal pathology
    - Neuromuscular disorders
    - Craniofacial disorders/Down syndrome
    - Upper respiratory infection w/in 4 weeks
    - Increased obstruction on induction
    - **OSA strong predictor of perioperative respiratory critical events**
- Management
    - **Extra caution when using a pre-med (benzo), increased risk apnea/hypopnea**
    - For minor, superficial surgeries, use regional anesthesia as much as possible
    - **Use minimal amount of opioids and try to use only short-acting**
    - Recommend alternatives to opioids (Tylenol, ketorolac, NSAIDS, local anesthetic, regional technique)
    - Be aware for possibility of difficult airway
    - Wake patient up completely, and make sure, if muscle relaxant used, that reversal is complete
    - If patient uses CPAP, make sure it is available for postoperative use
- Anticipate that patient may have to be admitted after surgery. Be vigilant in PACU and have a low threshold for admission.

Laryngospasm

- Definition: involuntary laryngeal closure, despite respiratory effort, airway emergency
- **Incidence: pediatric >>> adult**
- M&M: Desaturation, bradycardia, pulmonary aspiration, negative pressure pulmonary edema
- Risk Factors: **upper respiratory infection,** reactive airway disease, eczema, ear/nose/throat surgery, exposure to cigarette smoke
- **Recognition = rate limiting step**, primary reason for pediatric anesthesia fellowship
- Pt may exhibit "rocking-type" motion breathing, chest and abdomen not in sink, partial laryngospasm may have stridorous sound, or no sound at all if completely obstructed
- Interventions:
    - Call for help
    - 100% O_2
    - Attempt CPAP + airway adjustments (oral airway, double jaw thrust, 2-person ventilation)
    - IV in place: give succinylcholine (0.5 – 1 mg/kg) +/- atropine
    - No IV: give IM succinylcholine (3 – 4 mg/kg) +/- atropine
    - Intubate and re-evaluate patient for surgery continuing
    - Bradycardia secondary to hypoxia= epinephrine
    - Cardiac Arrest, follow PALS algorithm

Chapter 11: Pharmacology

- ❖ Quick Facts: Review of Pediatric Pharmacology Concepts
- ❖ Codeine
- ❖ Ketorolac
- ❖ Succinylcholine
- ❖ Propofol
- ❖ Propofol Infusion Syndrome
- ❖ Morphine
- ❖ Drug Bioavailability
- ❖ Medications with Black Box Warning for Pediatric Patients
- ❖ Commonly Used Drugs with Pediatric Dosage

Quick Facts: Review of Pediatric Pharmacology Concepts

- Increased volume of distribution = increased induction dose (increased TBW), particularly H_2O-soluble medication
- Decreased metabolism due to immature liver
- Decreased excretion due to immature kidney, decreased GFR
- Decreased protein binding = increased free medication, lowers threshold for toxicity
- Decreased fat/muscle = increased blood concentration of medication which would normally be taken up by fat/muscle

Codeine

- Naturally occurring weak mu-receptor prodrug
  - Potency that is approximately $1/10^{th}$ that of morphine
- The dose for all three routes (oral/IM/rectal) is 0.5 – 1.5 mg/kg
  - No longer given IV due to severe cardiopulmonary depression and seizures
- Most undergoes metabolism in the liver, some by CYP2D6 system
- Metabolite = morphine
- There are three major polymorphisms of this system:
  - Poor metabolizers (PM) results in no morphine, no pain relief
  - Extensive metabolizers (EM) produce normal amounts of morphine
  - **Ultra-extensive metabolizers (UM) produce rapid and large amounts of morphine, possible overdose**
- Greater amount of children are PM than originally thought.

Ketorolac

- Dose is usually 0.5 – 1 mg/kg q 6 hr IV, with max dose of 15 mg for children.
- Analgesic properties similar to low dose morphine
- Adverse effects
  - Reversible inhibition of platelet function - increased bleeding time
  - Bone healing in spinal fusion - high dosages
  - Can cause renal injury, caution with pts <1 year old
- Contraindications:
  - Patients with complete or partial syndrome of nasal polyps, angioedema, and bronchospastic reactivity
  - Renal dysfunction
  - GI bleed, GI ulcer disease
  - Major surgical procedure

Succinylcholine

- Depolarizing neuromuscular blocking drug
- IV doses
    - 1.5 – 2 mg/kg will depress twitches by 95% within 40 sec
    - 1 mg/kg will achieve the same in 50 sec
    - Infants younger than 1 year may need 3 mg/kg
- Infants more resistant to effects than adults (immature receptors, decreased muscle mass)
    - No fasiculations
- Tachyphylaxis
    - Generally develops after administration of 3 mg/kg
    - Phase II block occurs during tachyphylaxis after 4 mg/kg
- IM doses
    - Complete paralysis is usually gained in about 1 – 2 min
    - Dose 4 mg/kg produces profound relaxation
- Be aware of cholinesterase deficiency
    - Heterozygous occurs 1:30 (slightly prolonged or undetected)
    - Homozygous atypical is 1:3000 (1 hour prolongation)
    - Homozygous silent (up to 8 hours).
- Side effects
    - **Bradycardia!** (Particularly after 2nd dose)
    - TMJ stiffness
    - Hyperkalemia - up to 1 mEq/L increase
    - Fasiculations (not seen in infants)
    - Increased intraocular pressures
    - Increased ICP
- **BLACK BOX WARNING**
    - **Hyperkalemic cardiac arrests primarily in children with undiagnosed Duchenne muscular dystrophy**
- Succinylcholine recommendations in pediatric patients:
    - Emergency intubation (RSI)
    - Airway emergency (laryngospasm)

Propofol

- GABA$_A$ receptor
- Can reduce incidence of PONV
- Consider TIVA for the following pts:
    - Emergence delirium, malignant hyperthermia risk, Duchenne muscular dystrophy, severe post-op nausea/vomiting
- Lipid-based formula, aseptic technique must be used
- FDA prescribing information - contraindication: use caution in patients with egg, peanut and soy allergies
    - Other studies show no evidence for these contraindications

Propofol Infusion Syndrome

- Prolonged infusion: 70 mcg/kg/min for >48 hours
- **Signs/ symptoms:**
    - **Bradycardia** + lipemic plasma
    - Severe metabolic acidosis, hyperkalemia
    - Profound myocardial instability
    - Rhabdomyolysis and/or myoglobinuria
    - Enlarged fatty liver
- 80% mortality rate
- Tx: early hemodialysis
- Propofol inhibits mitochondrial respiration
- Predisposing risks: critically ill pts requiring catecholamine infusion, or high dose steroids
- Patients with fatty acid metabolism disorders may have increased risk

Morphine

- Most commonly used opioid
- Clearance of intravenous morphine similar to adult ranges by three months old
- Reduced clearance and prolonged $t_{1/2}$ in neonates
- Clearance: children > adults >>> neonates
- LD_{50} significantly reduced in neonates 2° immature blood brain barrier
- Extreme caution when used in infants < 1 year old
- Caution: histamine release = hypotension, urticaria = local response

Drug Bioavailability

Route	Percentage
Intravenous	1.0
Intramuscular	0.9
Intranasal	0.57
Rectal	0.4 – 0.5*
Oral	0.3*

*1st pass effect, extensive hepatic extraction

Medications with Black Box Warning for Pediatric Patients

- Succinylcholine – in Duchenne muscular dystrophy: lethal hyperkalemic cardiac arrest
- Codeine – in ultra-rapid metabolizers of CYP2D6: respiratory arrest
- Ketorolac – "not indicated for use in pediatric patients"
    - "Limited information available", translation no studies performed
- Note: Although there is no black box warning, dexmedetomidine is not FDA approved for pediatric use

Commonly Used Drugs and Pediatric Dosage

Resuscitation (given IV/IO unless otherwise noted)

Atropine	IV: 10-20 mcg/kg IV
	IM/PO: 20-30 mcg/kg IM
Calcium chloride	Arrest: 10 mg/kg
Epinephrine	Arrest: 10 mcg/kg IV/ETT
	Vasopressor: 0.5-5 mcg/kg IV
	Infusion: 0.02 - 1 mcg/kg/min IV
	Nebulizer: Racemic 2.25% solution 0.25-0.5 ml
Flumazenil	0.01 mg/kg (max 1 mg)
Intralipid	1-2 ml/kg of 20% emulsion
Lidocaine	1-2 mg/kg
Naloxone	Opioid overdose: 1-10 mcg/kg IV
	Opioid intoxication: 10 mcg/kg (max 2 mg)
Sodium Bicarbonate	1-2 mEq/kg

Antibiotics for Infective Endocarditis

Standard:	Amoxicillin	50 mg/kg (max 2 gm)
	Cefazolin	50 mg/kg (max 1 gm)
	Ampicillin	50 mg/kg (max 2 gm)
	Ceftriaxone	50 mg/kg (max 1 gm)
PCN allergy:	Clindamycin	20 mg/kg (max 600 mg)
	Cefazolin	50 mg/kg (max 2 gm)
MRSA+	Vancomycin	20 mg/kg (max 1 gm)

Antibiotics – Initial dose and 24 Hour dosing (IV)

Drug	Initial Dose	24 hr dose	Interval (h)
Ampicillin	50 mg/kg	100-400 mg/kg max 12 gm	Q4-6
Cefazolin	25-50 mg/kg	50-100 mg/kg max 12 gm	Q6-8
Cefotetan	40 mg/kg	40-80 mg/kg max 6 gm	Q12
Cefoxitin	40 mg/kg	80-160 mg/kg max 12 gm	Q6-8
Cefuroxime	25-50 mg/kg	75-150 mg/kg max 6-9 gm	Q6
Ciprofloxacin	10 mg/kg	20-30 mg/kg max 800 mg	Q12
Clindamycin	10-15 mg/kg	25-40 mg/kg max 1800 mg	Q6-8
Gentamicin	1.5-2.5 mg/kg	6-7.5 mg/kg	Q8-12
Metronidazole	15 mg/kg	30 mg/kg max 4 gm	Q6
Oxacillin	25 mg/kg	100-200 mg/kg max 12 gm	Q6
Vancomycin	10-15 mg/kg	40 mg/kg max 2 gm	Q8-12

MEDICATIONS (all IV/IO unless noted otherwise)

3% Sodium Chloride (Normal saline)	Hyponatremia Si/Sx - Infusion: 6 cc/kg over 1 hr increases Na^+ level by 5 mEq/L
Acetaminophen (Tylenol, Ofirmev))	PO: 10-15 mg/kg, max 75 mg/d IV: 15 mg/kg Q6 < 10 kg, 10mg/kg
Adenosine (Adenoscan, Adenocard)	0.1 mg/kg then 0.2 mg/kg
Albuterol	NEB: 0.15 mg/kg/dose (min 2.5 - 10mg) in 2 cc NS Continuous: 0.5 mg/kg/hr (max 15)
Alfentanil (Alfenta)	IV bolus: 10-50 mcg/kg Infusion: 1-3 mcg/kg/min IV
Aminocaproic acid (Amicar)	CPB: 100 mg/kg bolus over 30 min and in prime then 30 mg/kg/hr Non CV: 100 mg/kg bolus then 10 mg/kg/hr
Aminophylline (Phyllocontin, Truphylline)	6-7 mg/kg load over 20 min 1 mg/kg/hr (use 0.8 if <2 or >9 yo)
Amiodarone (Cordarone)	5 mg/kg; 5-10 mcg/kg/min
Amitriptyline	> 12 yo: start 10-25 mg/day (max 50-150 mg/day)
Atracurium (Tracrium)	0.5 mg/kg
Caffeine	20 mg/kg IV (as caffeine citrate) OR 10 mg/kg IV (as caffeine base)
Chloral hydrate	50-100 mg/kg PO/PR (max 2 g)
Chlorothiazide (Diuril)	10-15 mg/kg PO Q12
Cisatracurium (Nimbex)	0.1-0.2 mg/kg Infusion: 1-3 mcg/kg/min
Clonidine (Catapres, Kapvay)	PO: 5 mcg/kg/d div QID Opioid withdrawal: 0.1 mg BID-QID, taper over 10 d
Codeine	0.5-1 mg/kg PO (max 60 mg)
Desmopressin (DDAVP) (4 mcg=16 IU)	Hemophilia: 0.3 mcg/kg IV slowly DI: 1-2 mcg IV/SQ Q 12hr or 1-10 mU/kg/hr VW dz: 0.3 mcg/kg IV 30 prior to procedure
Dexamethasone (Decadron)	Airway edema: 0.25-0.5 mg/kg IV Q6hr ICP: 0.5-1.5 mcg/kg then 0.2-0.5 mg/kg/day Antiemetic: 0.1 mg/kg
Dexmedetomidine (Precedex)	Bolus: 0.2-2 mcg/kg over 10-20 min Infusion: 0.2-1 mcg/kg/hr
Dextrose	0.5 gm/kg = 1 cc/kg of D50
Diazepam (Valium, Diastat)	PO: 0.25-0.5 mg/kg (max 20 mg) IV: 0.1 mg/kg/dose
Diphenhydramine (Benadryl)	0.5-1 mg/kg IV/PO Q4-6 hr (max 50 mg) Anaphylaxis: 1-2 mg/kg

Dobutamine	2-20 mcg/kg/min
Docusate (Colace, Dulcolax)	<3 y: 10-40 mg/d; 3-6y: 20-60 mg/d 6-12 y: 40-120 mg/kg
Dopamine	2-20 mcg/kg/min
Droperidol (Ianpsine)	IM or IV: 0.1 mg/kg
Epinephrine	SC:(1:100) 0.01 cc/kg (max 0.5 cc/dose) Racemic: 2.25% sol; 0.25-0.5 ml via neb
Epinephrine	0.03-1 mcg/kg/min
Esmolol (Brevibloc)	0.1-0.5 mg/kg; 50-150 mcg/kg/min
Etomidate (Amidate)	0.2-0.6 mg/kg IV
Factor VIIa (Novoseven)	90 mcg/kg Q2hr until hemostasis
Factor VIII	1 u/kg raises plasma level 2%
Factor IX	1 u/kg raises level 1%
Fentanyl	IV: 0.5-2 mcg/kg Infusion 1-5 mcg/kg/hr
Fosphenytoin	20 mg PE/kg IV at 150 mg PE/min 1.5 mg fosphenytoin = 1mg phenytoin = 1 mg PE
Furosemide (Lasix)	0.5-1 mg/kg/dose IV Q6-12hr
Gabapentin	Start: 10-15 mg/kg/day titrated up Goal: 10-15 mg/kg/dose TID in < 60 kg pt Adult: max 3600 mg/day titrated up
Glucagon	0.1 mg/kg IV (max 1 mg)
Glycopyrrolate	0.01 mg/kg (max 1 mg)
Granisetron	10 mcg/kg (max 1 mg; PONV 0.1 mg)
Humate P (fVIII + vWF)	F8 deficiency: 40-60 u/kg then 20-30 u/kg IV Q8hr vWF deficiency: 40-80 u/kg IV then 40-60 u/kg Q8hr (types 2&3) or Q24hr (type 1)
Hydrocodone-acetaminophen (Lortab elixir)	5 ml =2.5 mg hydrocodone/167 mg acetaminophen 0.2 ml/kg Q4-6hr PO prn
Hydrocortisone (Solucortef)	Stress dose: 1-2 mg/kg IV then 150-250 mg/day (<1 y: 25-150 mg/d) divided Q6-8
Hydromorphone (Dilaudid)	IV: 5-10 mcg/kg IV PO/PR: 50-80 mcg/kg Q3-6hr prn
Hydroxyzine (Vistaril)	50-100 mg/day divided Q6-8hr PO
Ibuprofen (Advil, Motrin, Caldolor)	10 mg/kg PO Q6hr (max 800 mg)
Insulin	DKA drip: 0.1 u/kg/hr
Ipratropium (Atrovent)	INH Child: 250 mcg INH Adolescent: 500 mcg

Isoproterenol (Isuprel)	0.1-1 mcg/kg/min
Ketamine (Ketalar)	IV Induction: 1-3 mg/kg IM Induction: 5-8 mg/kg IM Sedation: 2-10mg/kg PO Sedation: 3-5 mg/kg
Ketorolac (Toradol)	0.5 mg/kg IV/IM Q6 (max 30 mg)
Labetalol	0.1-5 mg/kg; 1-3 mg/kg/hr
Lidocaine	1-2 mg/kg 20-40 mcg/kg/min
Lorazepam (Ativan)	IV: 0.1 mg/kg PR: 0.3 mg/kg IV/IM/PO Sedation: 0.05 mg/kg/dose (max 2 mg)
Magnesium sulfate	30 mg/kg
Mannitol	0.25-1 g/kg IV slowly Maintenance 0.25-0.5 g/kg IV Q4-6hr
Meperidine	0.5-2 mg/kg IV/IM
Methadone	0.05-0.1 mg/kg PO/IM/IV Q6-12
Methohexital	IV: 0.5-1 mg/kg PR: 25-30 mg/kg (max 600 mg)
Methylprednisolone (Solumedrol)	1 mg/kg IV initially, then 2 mg/kg/day divided Q4-6hr
Metoclopramide (Reglan)	IV/PO: 0.1-0.15 mg/kg Q6 hr prn
Midazolam	PO: 0.5-1 mg/kg (max 20 mg) IV: 0.1-0.2 mg/kg; 0.05-0.2 mg/kg/hr IM: 0.25 mg/kg Nasal: 0.2-0.3 mg/kg (max 10 mg) with atomizer
Milrinone	Load: 25-50 mcg/kg over 15 min Maintenance: 0.25-1 mcg/kg/min
Morphine	IV/IM: 0.05-0.1 mg/kg PO: 0.2-0.5 mg/kg/dose Q4-6 hr
Nalbuphine	0.05-0.1 mg/kg IV
Naloxone	IV: 1-10 mcg/kg for resp. depression (max 2 mg) Infusion: 2.5 -160 mcg/kg/hr
Neostigmine	0.03-0.07 mg/kg (max 5 mg)
Nicardipine (Cardene)	0.5-5 mcg/kg/min
Nitroprusside	0.5-20 mcg/kg/min
Norepinephrine	0.05-1 mcg/kg/min
Ondansetron (Zofran)	0.15 mg/kg IV max 4 mg
Oxycodone (Oxycontin)	PO: 0.05-0.15 mg/kg Q3-6hr prn

Pancuronium	0.05-0.1 mg/kg
Pentobarbital	1-6 mg/kg IV
Phenobarbitol	20 mg/kg IV; then 5 mg/kg Q2min (max 30 mg/kg)
Phenylephrine	0.5-1 mcg/kg 0.1-0.5 mcg/kg/min
Phenytoin (Dilantin)	20 mg/kg IV over 20 min
Potassium	0.5-1 mEq/kg slow IV infusion- central access preferred
Pregabalin (Lyrica)	PO: >12 yo: start 25-75 mg QHS (max 300 mg BID)
Procainamide	5-15 mg/kg; 20-80 mcg/kg/min
Prochlorperazine (Compazine)	0.1-0.15 mg/kg Q6-8 hr IV/PO/PR/IM (Max = 10 mg)
Promethazine (Phenergan)	0.25-0.5 mg/kg Q6-8 hr IV/PO/PR/IM Max = 25 mg/dose (not < 2 yo)
Propofol (Diprivan)	2-3 mg/kg IV Infusion: 50-250 mcg/kg/min
Prostaglndin E1	0.05-0.2 mcg/kg/min
Ranitidine (Zantac)	IV: 1 mg/kg PO: 2-5 mg/kg
Remifentanil (Ultiva)	IV bolus: 0.5-1 mcg/kg IV infusion: 0.05-0.5 mcg/kg/min
Rocuronium (Zemuron)	0.6 mg/kg 1.2 mg/kg (rapid sequence dose)
Scopolamine	0.02 mg/kg IV max 0.4 mg
Spironolactone	PO: 1 mg/kg Q8-12
Succinylcholine	1-2 mg/kg IV, 3-4 mg/kg IM
Sufentanil (Sufenta)	Analgesia: 0.5-2 mcg/kg IV Total dose: 10-20 mcg/kg
Terbutaline	NEB: 0.1 mg/kg in 2 cc NS (max 2.5 mg) IV: 5-10 mcg/kg load (max 250 mcg) over 20 min then 0.5-6 mcg/kg/min
Thiopental	4-8 mg/kg
Tramadol (Ultram)	1-2 mg/kg (max 50 mg) Q6hr
Transexamic Acid	100 mg/kg load; 10 mg/kg/hr
Vasopressin	0.3-2 milliunits/kg/min DI: 0.5-10 milliunits/kg/hr
Vecuronium	0.1 mg/kg

Chapter 12: Questions

1. During an exploratory laparotomy on a 2-month-old patient the $ETCO_2$ suddenly decreases to zero; EKG shows a sinus rhythm at 30 beats per minute, a pulse is not palpable. CPR with chest compressions is initiated. The PALS algorithm for pulseless electrical activity includes epinephrine to be given intravenously at the following dose?

    A. 0.1 mg/kg
    B. 0.01 mg/kg
    C. 0.001 mg/kg
    D. 0.0001 mg/kg

2. During a routine inhalation mask induction of an otherwise healthy 3-year-old boy, the patient is observed to have a rocking-type movement of his chest and abdomen, the oxygen saturation has rapidly decreased below 40% at this time. Attempts at positive pressure ventilation with an oral airway in place are unsuccessful. The immediate next step in clinical management should be to:

    A. Give intramuscular succinylcholine
    B. Place an LMA
    C. Place nasal trumpet
    D. Start an intravenous line

3. Inhalation mask induction is routine in healthy infants. The rapid onset, and therefore limited time in Stage II of anesthesia, is most likely attributed to which of the following?

    A. Decreased blood:gas solubility
    B. Decreased minute ventilation
    C. Increased cardiac output
    D. Increased minimum alveolar concentration

4. Of the following congenital cardiac defects, which occurs with the highest frequency?

    A. Atrial septal defect
    B. Coarctation of the aorta
    C. Transposition of the great arteries
    D. Ventricular septal defect

5. Necrotizing enterocolitis is increasingly successfully treated in the NICU. A perforated bowel would typically result in a surgical intervention. Which of the following abnormalities is most likely on a neonate with a perforated bowel?

    A. Alkalosis
    B. Hyperglycemia
    C. Hypervolemia
    D. Thrombocytopenia

6. Which of the following drugs has a black box warning specific for use in pediatric patients?

    A. Dantrolene
    B. Demerol
    C. Morphine
    D. Succinylcholine

7. With regards to the above question. Which of the following diseases/medical conditions is the responsible for the black box warning?

    A. Duchenne muscular dystrophy
    B. Malignant hyperthermia
    C. Respiratory arrest
    D. Sinus bradycardia

8. The incidence (number of cases per 1000) of malignant hyperthermia is_____ in the pediatric population vs adults.

    A. Decreased
    B. Increased
    C. Not reported
    D. The same

9. **Matching:** Disease with inheritance pattern, answers may be used more than once

    ____ Duchenne muscular dystrophy   A. Autosomal dominant
    ____ Malignant hyperthermia   B. Autosomal recessive
    ____ Hemophilia A   C. Random genetic mutation
    ____ Cystic fibrosis   D. X-linked recessive

10. In malignant hyperthermia a mutation in the coding of the ryanodine receptor is responsible for the abnormal muscle response to certain pharmacological triggers (succinylcholine, volatile anesthetics). The coding for the ryanodine receptor is found on which of the following chromosomes, in the majority of inherited malignant hyperthermia-susceptible individuals?

    A. Chromosome #19
    B. Chromosome #20
    C. Chromosome #21
    D. Chromosome #23

11. Of the following, which is the most likely presenting clinical sign of malignant hyperthermia?

    A. Hypertension
    B. Increased ETCO$_2$
    C. Tachypnea
    D. Tachycardia

12. You are covering the MRI suite for the day. A 7-day-old, full term baby arrives from outpatient for a brain MRI. The patient's history includes a diagnosis of intrauterine stroke. The baby was discharged from the hospital two days after birth, with no other signs or symptoms. Of the following, what would be the best course of action with regards to the scheduled procedure?

    A. Plan for a general anesthetic, mask induction followed by endotracheal intubation
    B. Plan for monitored anesthetic care with a propofol infusion
    C. Postpone MRI until patient is beyond one month of age
    D. Proceed with case, plan to admit to hospital post MRI

13. The spinal cord of a neonate typically extends to

    A. L1
    B. L2
    C. L3
    D. L4

14. You are caring for a 6-month-old healthy infant scheduled for a circumcision. After induction of general anesthesia and placement of an endotracheal tube, you prep and drape the patient for a caudal block. The procedure is initiated and the caudal space is found easily with successful "pop" appreciated as the needle pierces the ligament. During the test dose you notice spiked T waves, on the EKG. Your next immediate action should include

    A. Administer 1 ml/kg 20% intralipid
    B. Administer 10 mg/kg calcium chloride
    C. Repeat test dose
    D. Withdraw needle, abort procedure

15. When comparing functional residual capacity (FRC) between neonates and adults, the neonates FRC on an ml/kg basis is considered:

    A. Decreased by 25%
    B. Decreased by 30%
    C. Increased
    D. The same

16. A p50 of 26 mmHg is the partial pressure of oxygen at which adult hemoglobin is considered 50% saturated utilizing the oxygen-hemoglobin dissociation curve. There are several medical conditions, and clinical presentations that can shift the dissociation curve to the right or the left. Of the following, which is considered a right-shift on the oxygen-hemoglobin dissociation curve?

    A. Hemoglobin A
    B. Decreased 2,3-DPG
    C. Hemoglobin F
    D. Sickle cell hemoglobin

17. You are caring for a 1-year-old in the cath lab who is presenting for a percutaneous closure of their patent ductus arteriosus. Your current monitors include: pulse oximetry, 5-lead EKG, $ETCO_2$, an arterial pressure line, and nasal temperature. After deployment of the coil to occlude the ductus, which of the following clinical changes do you anticipate?

    A. Increased diastolic pressure
    B. Increased end tidal carbon dioxide concentration
    C. Increased oxygen saturation
    D. Increased temperature

18. The landmark bone structures for a caudal block are the sacral cornu which lie at the apex of the sacrum. Between the two cornu is the sacral hiatus which is covered by a ligament. This ligament provides the "pop" sensation when performing a caudal block. Which of the following is the correct ligament?

    A. Dorsal sacroiliac ligament
    B. Ligamentum flavum
    C. Posterior sacroiliac ligament
    D. Sacrococcygeal ligament

19. You have been called for a consult in the emergency room. The patient is 16 months old, presenting three days post-op following a circumcision. At present he is febrile, tachycardic, irritable, and the parents report "swelling and redness" above the buttocks. The patient had an uneventful general anesthetic in addition to a caudal block. The most valuable next step in diagnosis at this time would be

    A. Consult Infectious Disease
    B. Order a CBC with differential
    C. Order an MRI scan
    D. Order an ultrasound

Questions #20 – 23 Matching: Difficult airway syndromes with characteristics

20. _____ Treacher Collins syndrome

21. _____ Pierre Robin syndrome

22. _____ Beckwith-Wiedemann syndrome

23. _____ Goldenhar Syndrome

    A. Unilateral hemifacial hypoplasia, absent ear
    B. Macroglossia, gigantism, hypoglycemia
    C. Mandibular hypoplasia, macrostomia, cleft palate
    D. Micrognathia, glossoptosis, respiratory distress

Questions # 24 – 28 refer to the following case scenario

An 11-year-old 41.8 kg female has been schedule with general anesthesia for chest tube placement. The patient reports a two month history of "new onset wheeze" for which she was treated with albuterol. She presented to an outside hospital for increasing respiratory difficulties and was transferred to your pediatric center after a chest x-ray was obtained. On exam the patient is resting comfortably sitting upright on a stretcher; she has reduced breath sounds on the left, and cannot lay supine without significantly labored breathing.

Vital signs: SpO_2 95% on room air, RR 29, temp is 37.2° C, HR is 135, BP is 126/89.
CXR: Large pleural effusions L>R, widened mediastinum

24. The likely diagnosis from a biopsy would reveal?

    A. Acute lymphoblastic leukemia
    B. Non-Hodgkin lymphoma
    C. Small cell carcinoma
    D. Wilms tumor

25. Based on the above information, what additional diagnostic test should be included in the patient's pre-operative workup?

    A. A PET scan
    B. An ECHO
    C. An MRI
    D. An ultrasound

26. The surgeon has requested a general anesthesia for the chest tube placement. What is the safest anesthetic technique for the above patient?

    A. A general anesthetic, IV induction with ketamine
    B. A general anesthetic, mask induction
    C. Monitored anesthesia care with a propofol infusion
    D. Placing chest tube with local anesthetic

27. It becomes necessary to perform general anesthesia with a mask induction for the chest tube placement. After an inhalation mask induction you are able to successfully intubate the patient, confirming with +$ETCO_2$, as well as bilateral breath sounds. At this time the surgeon requests relaxation and you administer 20 mg rocuronium IV. Seconds after flushing the rocuronium, you notice peak pressures have increased to 45 cm H_2O, tidal volumes have decreased to 60 ml, and pulse oxygen saturation has started to drop. The next immediate intervention should be?

    A. Give glycopyrrolate and neostigmine in rapid succession
    B. Place a needle at the 2nd intercostal space
    C. Place patient in lateral decubitus position
    D. Reconfirm ETT position

28. In a patient with an anterior mediastinal mass, which of the following is MOST indicative of a high incidence of complications perioperatively?

    A. Bilateral pleural effusions
    B. Mediastinal widening on chest X-ray
    C. Peak expiratory flow rate <10% of predicted
    D. Tracheal compression >50% on CT scan

29. Which of the following would not typically be expected in a patient with VACTERL syndrome?

    A. Anal atresia
    B. Choanal atresia
    C. Radial atresia
    D. Vertebral anomalies

30. Which one of the following DECREASES pulmonary vascular resistance?

    A. Acidosis
    B. Hypercarbia
    C. Prostaglandin E1
    D. Prostaglandin F2

31. EMLA cream is commonly used in pediatrics as a topical anesthetic for intravenous placement. EMLA cream contains a mixture of two local anesthetics. Which is the correct pairing?

    A. Lidocaine and mepivacaine
    B. Lidocaine and tetracaine
    C. Lidocaine and procaine
    D. Lidocaine and prilocaine

32. Which of the following patients requires a higher ml/kg/min perfusion pressure during cardiopulmonary bypass?

    A. 2-week-old male
    B. 2-year-old male
    C. 12-year-old female
    D. 60-year-old male

33. When caring for a Moyamoya patient during a procedure that requires a general anesthetic, which of the following situations is known to potentiate significant morbidity, and should be avoided?

    A. High inspired oxygen concentration
    B. Hypercarbia
    C. Hypocarbia
    D. Hypoventilation

34. Inhaled nitric oxide, a treatment for pulmonary hypertension, is metabolized quickly via oxidation at which of the following sites?

    A. Kidney
    B. Liver
    C. Plasma
    D. Red blood cell

35. The head of a neonate comprises approximately what percent of its body surface area?

    A. 9%
    B. 10%
    C. 18%
    D. 25%

36. Which of the following is likely to increase right to left shunting in a patient with tetralogy of Fallot?

    A. 10 ml/kg crystalloid bolus
    B. Crying
    C. Increased systemic vascular resistance
    D. 100% inspired oxygen

37. Brown fat is present in neonates and is responsible for "non-shivering" thermogenesis. Metabolism of brown fat results in heat production for the neonate and subsequently heat loss. Brown fat is highly vascular and has predominately which of the following innervation?

    A. A-delta fibers
    B. A-gamma fibers
    C. C fibers
    D. β-sympathetic fibers

38. Calculate the protamine dose required, if pre-bypass heparin dose was 6,000 units.

    A. 6 mg
    B. 60 mg
    C. 600 mg
    D. 6,000 mg

39. Of the following, which is expected to be naturally elevated in a healthy one month old infant?

    A. Bicarbonate
    B. Blood urea nitrogen
    C. Glucose
    D. Potassium

Questions #40 and #41 refer to the following case scenario

You are caring for an otherwise healthy 14-year-old female, who is under general anesthesia for a cosmetic plastics procedure. Medications given for induction include: midazolam, fentanyl, propofol and rocuronium. Following intubation, clindamycin was given as the requested antibiotic. At this time the ventilator begins to alarm; you note peak airway pressures have increased from 15 to 40 cm H_2O, patient is also tachycardic, pulse oxygen saturation is in the low 80s, and the patient appears to have a flushed appearance on her head and neck.

40. The top of your differential diagnosis should be:

    A. Anaphylaxis
    B. Mucous plug
    C. Pulmonary embolus
    D. Tension pneumothorax

41. After reconfirming correct placement of your endotracheal tube, you note diminished air movement bilaterally, the patient's pulse oxygen saturation is presently 85%, heart rate 135, and current blood pressure 70/35 mmHg. Your next immediate intervention should include:

    A. Ephedrine
    B. Epinephrine
    C. Needle decompression in the 2nd left intercostal space
    D. Phenylephrine

42. PGE 1 (prostaglandin) is commonly used in selected congenital heart defects to maintain the patency of the ductus arteriosus. Which is typically not considered a "ductal-dependent" lesion?

    A. Critical coarctation of aorta
    B. Pulmonary atresia
    C. Transposition of the great arteries
    D. Ventricular septal defect

43. Working in the MRI suite requires knowledge of the specific safety concerns related to the magnetic field created by the MRI. There are "MRI-compatible" oxygen and nitrous tanks available. These MRI-compatible gas tanks contain the following non-magnetic metals:

    A. Aluminum
    B. Iron
    C. Nickel
    D. Steel

44. Of the following volatile anesthetics, which has the lowest percentage of metabolism?

    A. Desflurane
    B. Halothane
    C. Isoflurane
    D. Sevoflurane

45. NPO duration for breast milk is?

    A. 2 hours
    B. 4 hours
    C. 6 hours
    D. 8 hours

46. All of the following congenital cardiac anomalies are associated with cyanosis except?

    A. Hypoplastic left heart
    B. Tetralogy of Fallot
    C. Tricuspid atresia
    D. Atrial septal defect

47. Epiglottitis is now a relatively rare infectious disease. The classic radiographic image shows:

    A. Deviated trachea
    B. Hyperinflation
    C. Steeple sign
    D. Thumbprint sign

48. You are caring for an otherwise healthy 2-year-old male, who is presently under general anesthesia for strabismus surgery. Procedure is well underway and vitals have been stable throughout. Without warning, there is an acute change in your patient's heart rate, with significant bradycardia, all other vitals remain at baseline. You suspect a common reflex. What is the afferent limb of this reflex?

    A. Cranial Nerve III
    B. Cranial Nerve V
    C. Cranial Nerve VI
    D. Cranial Nerve X

49. During a surgical procedure for ligation of a patent ductus arteriosus, injury to the left recurrent laryngeal nerve is possible. Which of the following is NOT innervated by the left recurrent laryngeal nerve?

    A. Cricothyroid muscle
    B. Lateral cricoarytenoid muscle
    C. Posterior cricoarytenoid muscle
    D. Thyroarytenoid muscle

Questions #50 – 53 refer to the following case scenario

An 8-week-old infant is scheduled for a laparoscopic pyloromyotomy procedure as the first case of the day. The patient was admitted yesterday and appropriately resuscitated with intravenous fluids. Lab work today is in normal range. While interviewing the mother, she reports the baby was fed formula just prior to coming to the pre-op holding area.

50. At this time the next course of action should be

    A. Postpone case for 4 hours, following NPO guidelines
    B. Postpone case for 6 hours, following NPO guidelines
    C. Proceed with case; it is an emergency
    D. Proceed with case; patient is considered a full stomach regardless of NPO status.

51. Pyloric stenosis occurs more frequently in males than females.

    A. True
    B. False

52. Presenting lab work on a patient with pyloric stenosis will likely show?

    A. Metabolic acidosis with hyperkalemia and hypochloremia
    B. Metabolic alkalosis with hyperkalemia and hyperchloremia
    C. Metabolic alkalosis with hypokalemia and hyperchloremia
    D. Metabolic alkalosis with hypokalemia and hypocholoremia

53. Induction of patients with pyloric stenosis requires skill and knowledge of the pathophysiology. Once in the operating room after monitors are on, you suction the stomach in three positions, pre-oxygenate your patient, and prepare for induction. Which of the following would not be a recommended induction technique for this patient?

    A. Awake intubation
    B. Mask induction with N_2O/O_2 and 8% sevoflurane
    C. Rapid sequence induction with rocuronium
    D. Rapid sequence induction with succinylcholine

54. Marfan syndrome, a connective tissue disorder, frequently leads to aortic root dilation. Another valve commonly affected is:

    A. Mitral valve
    B. Pulmonary valve
    C. Tricuspid valve
    D. Typically only the aortic valve is affected

55. A junctional rhythm implies the loss of AV synchronicity. An EKG will show a loss of P waves, or even a retrograde P wave, however this is often difficult to discern with concurrent tachycardia. One way to confirm the junctional rhythm is with a central venous catheter tracing, which will show which of the following?

    A. Dampening of all wave forms
    B. Decreased a waves
    C. Decreased v waves
    D. Increased v waves

56. You are preparing to perform a caudal block on an otherwise healthy 5-month-old, 7 kg male for a scheduled circumcision. You plan to use 0.25% bupivacaine with 1:200,000 epinephrine as your local anesthetic for the caudal block. Please calculate your patient's maximum allowed dosage of the local anesthetic for the above listed concentration.

    A. 7 mg
    B. 17.5 mg
    C. 21 mg
    D. 49 mg

57. An inhalation mask induction would theoretically take longer for which of the following congenital cardiac anomalies?

    A. Atrial septal defect
    B. Coarctation of the aorta
    C. Pulmonary atresia
    D. Ventricular septal defect

58. Which of the following patients do you anticipate to have the highest volume of cerebral spinal fluid on an ml/kg basis?

    A. Preterm infant
    B. Term infant
    C. 5-year-old
    D. 25-year-old

59. Bupivacaine at 0.125% concentration contains how many milligrams per milliliter?

    A. 0.0125 mg/ml
    B. 0.125 mg/ml
    C. 1.25 mg/ml
    D. 12.5 mg/ml

60. You are scheduled to care for a healthy 2-month-old patient, for a cleft lip repair. Your anesthetic plan includes general anesthesia in addition to an infraorbital nerve block. The infraorbital nerve is a branch of the following?

    A. V_1 - ophthalmic division
    B. V_2 - maxillary division
    C. V_3 - mandibular division
    D. X - vagus

61. Cleft lip is more common in females than males.

    A. True
    B. False

62. Cleft lip is more common on the left side than the right side.

    A. True
    B. False

63. Which of the following syndromes which has the highest association with cleft lip and cleft palate?

    A. Klippel-Feil syndrome
    B. Pierre Robin syndrome
    C. Treacher Collins syndrome
    D. Velocardiofacial syndrome

Questions #64 and #65 refer to the following case scenario

A 5-year-old female is scheduled for a routine surveillance MRI of the brain. The patient is currently receiving treatment for a primary brain tumor, medical history is otherwise unremarkable. Parents deny cough, cold or recent fever. After a smooth intravenous induction and uneventful LMA placement, bilateral breath sounds are confirmed and positive end tidal carbon dioxide is appreciated. Despite 100% inspired oxygen and clear breath sounds, the pulse oximetry saturation is 85%.

64. Based on the above description you suspect which of the following clinical scenarios to explain the hypoxia?

    A. Bronchospasm
    B. Methemoglobinemia
    C. Mucous plug
    D. Oxygen supply line crossed over with air

65. After confirming breath sounds are clear and equal, you suspect which of the following agents could explain the hypoxia unresponsive to oxygen?

    A. Adriamycin
    B. Bleomycin
    C. Cisplatin
    D. Dapsone

66. Patients with increased predisposition to obstructive sleep apnea include:

    A. Down syndrome
    B. Goldenhar syndrome
    C. Pierre Robin syndrome
    D. All of the above

67. _____ management for cardiopulmonary bypass is a method of monitoring blood gases correcting for the actual body temperature and increasing pH to 7.40 and $PaCO_2$ to 40.

    A. Alpha-STAT
    B. pH-STAT

68. In a patient with unrepaired tetralogy of Fallot, which of the following induction agents would you anticipate to have the slowest onset?

    A. Halothane
    B. Ketamine
    C. Propofol
    D. Sevoflurane

103

69. Which of the following diseases is not considered susceptible to malignant hyperthermia?

    A. Central core disease
    B. Duchenne muscular dystrophy
    C. King-Denborough disease
    D. Multiminicore disease

70. Dantrolene must be reconstituted at the time of delivery with which of the following:

    A. D_5W solution
    B. Lactated Ringers solution
    C. Normal saline solution
    D. Preservative free water

71. The theoretical improvement in neurological outcomes in infants post cardiopulmonary bypass that were managed on bypass with pH-Stat for arterial blood gases is believed to be from:

    A. Decreased emboli
    B. Decreased $PaCO_2$
    C. Increased blood viscosity
    D. Increased cerebral blood flow

72. An intensive care patient presents for a G-tube placement. The patient is 4 months old this week and was born at 25 weeks gestation. Please calculate the patients post gestational age (PGA).

    A. 16 weeks
    B. 29 weeks
    C. 41 weeks
    D. 55 weeks

73. Post-operative tonsillectomy hemorrhage is a serious complication, with significant risk for morbidity and mortality. The majority of these cases occur

    A. Post-operative day #7
    B. Post-operative hemorrhage is virtually unheard of
    C. Within 6 hours of surgery
    D. Within 24 hours of surgery

74. A 6-year-old patient has returned to the emergency department post-operatively, following a tonsillectomy and adenoidectomy. The surgeon has requested to take the patient to the operating room immediately. The recommended induction plan for this case would be?

    A. Awake fiberoptic induction
    B. Inhalation mask induction
    C. Intramuscular induction
    D. Rapid sequence induction

75. An 8-year-old patient is scheduled for an emergent exploratory laparotomy for suspected bowel perforation. The patient's abdominal X-ray shows free air under the diaphragm. Patient is resuscitated in the emergency room with two liters of normal saline.
    Vital signs: HR 150, BP 70/30, RR 30, Temp 38.5°C
    Labs: Hb/Hct 7/25, ABG: pH 7.1
    Of the following medications which would be the best choice for the induction of general anesthesia?

    A. Fentanyl
    B. Ketamine
    C. Propofol
    D. Sevoflurane

76. A 3 year old patient with a secundum type atrial septal defect has a Qp:Qs ratio of 2:1. Which of the following is understood by this Qp:Qs ratio?

    A. Mean pulmonary artery pressure 2X normal
    B. Pulmonary artery blood flow 2X systemic blood flow
    C. Pulmonary vascular resistance 2X normal
    D. Right atrial pressure 2X normal

77. A 15-month-old patient presents for an airway foreign body removal. The foreign body is believed to be a peanut. Which of the following is a recommended goal for your anesthetic management?

    A. Awake intubation
    B. Maintain spontaneous ventilation
    C. Muscle relaxation
    D Rapid sequence induction

78. In order for cyanosis to be observed in a patient clinically, what is the minimum concentration of hemoglobin (g/dL)?

    A. 5
    B. 10
    C. 15
    D. 20

79. Which of the following is a common co-morbidity in a healthy newborn with Beckwith-Wiedemann syndrome?

    A. Gastroschesis
    B. Hydrocephalus
    C. Imperforate anus
    D. Omphalocele

80. In a newborn with meconium ileus which disease must be ruled out?

    A. Cystic fibrosis
    B. Duchene muscular dystrophy
    C. Sickle cell disease
    D. Tay-Sachs

81. The age group with the highest percent of fatalities from child abuse is:

    A. <1 year old
    B. 1 year old
    C. 2 year old
    D. 3 year old

82. You have just performed a deep extubation on a 2-year-old patient at completion of an uneventful upper endoscopy exam. After placing the oxygen mask on your patient you notice you no longer have end tidal carbon dioxide, you attempt positive pressure ventilation, in addition to an oral airway with no improvement. The patient's oxygen saturation is rapidly decreasing, and bradycardia with a heart rate of 30 is noted. You suspect complete laryngospasm and give succinylcholine intravenously, your next intervention at this time should be:

    A. Atropine
    B. Albuterol via mask
    C. Chest compressions
    D. Glycopyrrolate

83. An ex-26-week premature infant is in the PACU. The PACU nurse calls to report a witnessed apneic event that responded to stimulation, but required blow by oxygen to recover oxygen saturations into the 90s. This patient was scheduled to be discharged following their procedure. What is the minimum time that this patient should be monitored, and apnea-free prior to discharge?

    A. 3 hours
    B. 6 hours
    C. 12 hours
    D. 24 hours

84. A general surgeon asks you to add a case to the schedule for tomorrow morning. The patient is a full term male infant, now 10 weeks old with a two week history of refractory projectile vomiting. The patient failed to gain weight at his last well check visit, and now appears lethargic, parents report no wet diaper in the last six hours. Which of the following results do you anticipate from his metabolic panel?

	Na^+	K^+	Cl^-	CO_2
A.	155	5.5	110	20
B.	140	4.0	100	25
C.	135	2.4	73	50
D.	140	2.5	96	29

85. Duodenal atresia is most commonly associated with which of the following syndromes?

    A. Down syndrome
    B. Sticklers syndrome
    C. Turner syndrome
    D. Williams syndrome

Questions # 86 – 89: Matching: Diagnosis with radiographic findings

86. ___ Necrotizing enterocolitis

87. ___ Duodenal atresia

88. ___ Congenital diaphragmatic hernia

89. ___ Pyloric stenosis

    A. Double bubble sign
    B. Free air under the diaphragm
    C. Intestines above diaphragm
    D. Olive-shaped mass

90. Which of the following is not a risk factor for obstructive sleep apnea?

    A. African American ethnicity
    B. Down syndrome
    C. Male
    D. Obesity

91. All of the following are signs/symptoms of a high spinal except:

    A. Apnea
    B. Dilated pupils
    C. Loss of consciousness
    D. Pinpoint pupils

92. A 2-year-old, 13 kg male presents for a tonsil and adenoidectomy. Calculate this patient's fluid deficit assuming eight hours NPO status.

    A. 320 ml
    B. 344 ml
    C. 368 ml
    D. 418 ml

93. A two-month-old patient with an unrepaired tetralogy of Fallot presents for repair of an incarcerated hernia. Which of the following anesthetics is recommended for the induction of general anesthesia for this patient?

    A. Ketamine
    B. Morphine
    C. Propofol
    D. Sevoflurane

94. A previously healthy 7-year-old male is to be taken emergently to your cath lab for a pericardial drainage. The patient presented with a large pericardial effusion, history is remarkable for three days of low grade fever, and "not feeling well". The ECHO shows a 3 cm effusion surrounding the heart, with significant ventricular compression. The patient is resting comfortably, however he is tachypneic, tachycardic, and his blood pressure is elevated for the patient's age. You are preparing to intubate the patient for the procedure. Which of the following would be the best option for your induction?

    A. Fentanyl
    B. Ketamine
    C. Propofol
    D. Sevoflurane

Questions #95 and #96 refer to the following case scenario

You are called emergently to help a colleague in the operating room. Upon arrival you note the surgeon is performing chest compressions, and the anesthesia resident tells you the patient does not have a pulse.

95. The EKG shows V-tach, pulse oximetry saturation shows no waveform or number value; you confirm there is no pulse. Your next immediate intervention should be:

    A. Prepare to intubate the patient
    B. Give intravenous amiodarone
    C. Give intravenous epinephrine
    D. Prepare to shock

96. While placing the defibrillating pads on the patient, the resident informs you that this is a 3-year-old, 15 kg male. For the initial shock, you request the request the defibrillator be charged to:

    A. 15 joules
    B. 30 joules
    C. 60 joules
    D. 200 joules

97. You are performing a caudal block on an otherwise healthy 8-month-old male for a circumcision. You have chosen 0.25% bupivacaine with 1:200,000 epinephrine for the block. After performing a test dose, which of the following would you likely see first, indicating a positive test dose?

    A. Increased heart rate greater than 10 beats/minute
    B. Increased systolic blood pressure greater than 15 mmHg
    C. Increased T waves
    D. Premature ventricular contractions

98. Normal resting intracranial pressure in an infant is elevated compared to an adult.

    A. True
    B. False

99. When comparing lung volume differences between infants and adults, which of the following volumes is decreased in an infant?

    A. Dead space (ml/kg)
    B. Functional residual capacity (ml/kg)
    C. Lung volumes are the same in infants and adults
    D. Total lung capacity (ml/kg)

100. Which of the following lung volumes is decreased in infants compared to adults?

    A. Closing volume
    B. Inspiratory reserve volume
    C. Residual volume
    D. All of the above

101. Of possible foreign bodies in the airway, the peanut has increased morbidity. Comparing an unroasted peanut to a roasted peanut, which has an increased inflammatory response?

    A. Inflammatory response equal
    B. No inflammatory response
    C. Roasted peanut
    D. Unroasted peanut

102. Which of the following are true in regards to effect of heart rate and stroke volume on neonatal cardiac output?

    A. Heart rate has greatest impact on cardiac output
    B. Neither heart rate or stroke volume impact cardiac output in a neonate
    C. Stroke volume and heart rate equally increase cardiac output
    D. Stroke volume has greatest impact on cardiac output

103. What is the estimated blood volume (EBV) of a neonate born at 32 weeks gestation, 1500 grams?

    A. 120 mL
    B. 127 mL
    C. 142 mL
    D. 200 mL

104. What is the risk of abruptly stopping total parental nutrition in a 34-week-old neonate scheduled for a 3 hour abdominal surgery?

    A. Direct hyperbilirubinemia
    B. Hypertriglyceridemia
    C. Hypoglycemia
    D. Sepsis

105. Compared to an adult, neonatal oxygen consumption, tidal volumes and respiratory rate differ in what way, respectively?

   A. Decreased, unchanged, decreased
   B. Decreased, increased, increased
   C. Increased, increased, increased
   D. Increased, unchanged, increased

106. The intensive care unit nurse calls for emergency airway help on a 1 kg newborn infant. Which size endotracheal tube would you most likely choose to intubate this patient?

   A. 2.0 mm
   B. 2.5 mm
   C. 3.0 mm
   D. 3.5 mm

107. You are called to assist with the airway management of a preterm infant with an intrauterine diagnosis of a left-sided congenital diaphragmatic hernia (CDH). The neonate has minimal respiratory effort and the heart rate is in the 50s. What is the most appropriate airway intervention?

   A. Blow-by oxygen
   B. Continuous positive airway pressure (CPAP)
   C. Intubate the trachea
   D. Positive pressure ventilation (PPV)

108. After pre-oxygenating a one-week-old infant, you perform an intravenous induction followed by endotracheal intubation. During intubation the patient's pulse oxygen saturation drops precipitously. Which of the following explains such a rapid oxygen desaturation?

   A. Increased O_2 consumption
   B. Increased functional residual capacity
   C. Increased total lung capacity
   D. None of the above

109. Which of the following is a triggering agent for malignant hyperthermia?

   A. Ketamine
   B. Nitrous oxide
   C. Rocuronium
   D. Succinylcholine

110. Which of the following is not considered an early clinical sign of malignant hyperthermia?

    A. Tachycardia
    B. Elevated temperature
    C. Tachypnea
    D. Increased end tidal carbon dioxide

111. Once malignant hyperthermia is suspected, what is the most important next clinical intervention?

    A. Give epinephrine
    B. Hyperventilate
    C. Treat tachycardia
    D. Discontinue triggering agent

112. An infant born at 32 weeks gestation and weighing 1.4 kg is scheduled for a liver biopsy for direct hyperbilirubinemia, hepatomegaly, and jaundice. Day of surgery coagulation lab results are as follows: INR 1.6, PTT 35.5, fibrinogen 65. Which would be most likely to correct these deficiencies?

    A. Cryoprecipitate
    B. Factor VII
    C. Fresh frozen plasma
    D. Platelets

113. Which of the following is not a component of cryoprecipitate?

    A. Factor VII
    B. Factor VIII
    C. Factor XIII
    D. Fibrinogen

114. Fresh frozen plasma and cryoprecipitate are interventions used for many disease processes. Which of the following diseases would be most likely to benefit from the factors present in cryoprecipitate?

    A. Antithrombin III deficiency
    B. Factor VII deficiency
    C. Hemophilia A
    D. Hemophilia B

115. You have been requested to place an arterial line via the umbilical artery in a newborn infant. Trace the path of an umbilical artery catheter as it is inserted.

    A. Umbilical artery - Common Iliac artery - Hypogastric artery - Aorta
    B. Hypogastric artery - Aorta - Umbilical artery - Common Iliac artery
    C. Umbilical artery - Hypogastric artery - Aorta - Common Iliac artery
    D. Umbilical artery - Hypogastric artery - Common Iliac artery - Aorta

116. A one-day-old neonate who was born at 36 weeks gestation is spontaneously breathing on room air and is cyanotic at rest but coloration and oxygenation improve when the infant is crying. What is the most likely diagnosis?

    A. Choanal atresia
    B. Persistent pulmonary hypertension of the newborn
    C. Normal finding in newborn
    D. Transient tachypnea of the newborn

117. A former 28-week-old neonate is now 18 months old. The child was intubated immediately after birth, and required long term ventilation which ultimately resulted in a tracheostomy. How would ventilator settings differ in this child at 18 months compared to shortly after birth?

    A. Decreased tidal volume
    B. Increase inspiratory time
    C. Increased respiratory rate
    D. None of the above

118. Which of the following causes a leftward shift in the oxygenation dissociation curve?

    A. Acidosis
    B. Fetal hemoglobin
    C. Hyperthermia
    D. Increased 2,3-diphosphoglycerate (DPG)

Questions #119 – 122 refer to the following case scenario

At 34 weeks gestation, a neonate was delivered emergently secondary to decreased heart rate variability in addition to late heart rate deceleration. Shortly after delivery, the neonate appeared cyanotic. Continuous positive airway pressure was applied with minimal improvement in oxygenation saturations. Pre and post-ductal oxygenation saturations were obtained.

119. Where would you place the pulse oximeters to obtain pre- and post-ductal oxygen saturations?

    A. Left hand and right foot
    B. Right hand and left ear
    C. Right hand and left foot
    D. Right hand and right ear

120. After placing the pulse oximeters, you note that the pre-ductal SpO_2 reads 90% and the post-ductal SpO_2 reads 70%. What does this gradient most likely indicate?

    A. Normal finding in a newborn
    B. Premature closure of the ductus arteriosus
    C. Significant left-to-right shunt
    D. Significant right-to-left shunt

121. An ECHO was ordered emergently which showed no structural abnormalities of the heart, and a normal shortening fraction. Based on this added information what is the most likely explanation for the oxygen saturation gradient in the above patient?

    A. Normal finding in newborn
    B. Persistent pulmonary hypertension of the newborn
    C. Respiratory distress syndrome
    D. Ischemia of the lower extremity

122. Which of the following interventions would you expect to limit a right-to-left shunt?

    A. Decrease pulmonary vascular resistance
    B. Increase preload
    C. Increase systemic vascular resistance
    D. All of the above

Questions #123-126 Matching:

123. ___ Tetralogy of Fallot

124. ___ Truncus arteriosus

125. ___ Total anomalous pulmonary venous return

126. ___ Ebstein anomaly

    A. "Box-shaped" heart on CXR
    B. "Boot-shaped" heart on CXR
    C. Figure of eight, "snowman" sign on CXR
    D. Significant cardiomegaly, right aortic arch

127. What changes on a high frequency oscillator (HFO) ventilator can be made to correct pCO_2?

    A. Amplitude
    B. Hertz
    C. Mean airway pressure
    D. A & B

128. What is the equivalent of "rate" on a high frequency oscillator ventilator?

    A. Amplitude
    B. Frequency
    C. Hertz
    D. Mean airway pressure

129. What clinical parameter do you use to determine adequacy of high frequency oscillator ventilator settings?

    A. Abdominal distention
    B. Breath sounds
    C. Chest rise
    D. Chest wiggle

130. A 2-year-old patient was on cardiopulmonary bypass (CPB) for 3 hours. After successfully weaning the patient from CPB, the surgeon requests protamine to be given. Which of the following are possible side effects of protamine?

    A. Coagulation abnormalities
    B. Pulmonary hypertension
    C. Systemic hypotension
    D. All of the above

Questions # 131-136 Matching: Pharmacology

131. ____ Epinephrine

132. ____ Dobutamine

133. ____ Milrinone

134. ____ Dopamine

135. ____ Isoproterenol

136. ____ Phenylephrine

   A. Can increase splanchnic and renal perfusion even at high doses.
   B. Good choice to augment contractility and perfusion, used in patient with compromised ventricular function or patients with anaphylaxis.
   C. Increases systemic vascular resistance, pure alpha agonist. Can cause significant reflex bradycardia.
   D. Positive inotropy and lusitropy by increasing cyclic adenosine monophosphate (cAMP).
   E. Pure, nonselective beta agonist. May be useful in children with bradycardia or post-heart transplant patients.
   F. Selective beta 1 (minimal beta 2) activity with side effects including tachycardia and vasodilation.

137. Which of the following agents used in the treatment of pulmonary hypertension is responsible for methemoglobinemia?

   A. Epoprostenol
   B. Inhaled nitric oxide
   C. Prostaglandin E1
   D. Sildenafil

138. A 3-month-old patient is undergoing surgery for correction of tetralogy of Fallot. Prior to cardiopulmonary bypass, heparin is given as 400 mg/kg intravenously. The follow-up ACT is less than 300 sec. A second bolus of heparin is given with similar ACT results. What should be considered at this time?

   A. Antithrombin III deficiency
   B. Faulty ACT reading
   C. Heparin induced thrombocytopenia
   D. Inadequate time for heparin to take effect

139. In an otherwise healthy term infant you can expect the patient's birth weight to increase by approximately how much at the age of six months?

    A. 10%
    B. 20%
    C. 50%
    D. 100%

140. An infant's first breath is important in developing their functional residual capacity (FRC). Nearly 50% of the first breath will be retained for their FRC. The first breath generated by a newborn develops approximately how much negative intrathoracic pressure?

    A. 20 cm H_2O
    B. 30 cm H_2O
    C. 60 cm H_2O
    D. 100 cm H_2O

141. Static lung volumes such as vital capacity and functional residual capacity are linearly related to a logarithm of

    A. Age
    B. Height
    C. Weight
    D. None of the above

142. There are multiple delivery routes for midazolam. Which of the following routes would you anticipate the fastest onset?

    A. Intramuscular
    B. Nasal
    C. Oral
    D. Rectal

143. In a patient with craniosynostosis, which of the following sutures is considered the most common site of premature closure?

    A. Coronal
    B. Lambdoidal
    C. Metopic
    D. Sagittal

144. An ECHO report for a one-year-old patient will likely report the "shortening fraction", as opposed to the "ejection fraction". The shortening fraction relies on which of the following parameters?

    A. Left ventricular end diastolic diameter
    B. Left ventricular end diastolic volume
    C. Left ventricular end systolic pressure
    D. Left ventricular end systolic volume

145. A 3-month-old patient is scheduled for repair of a ventricular septal defect. Which of the following VSD types is the most common?

    A. Inlet
    B. Muscular
    C. Perimembranous
    D. Sub-arterial

146. A two-month-old infant has a large unrestricted ventricular septal defect, which of the following is most likely?

    A. Cyanosis
    B. Hypertension
    C. Increased hematocrit
    D. Pulmonary vascular congestion

147. Prostaglandin E1, alprostadil, is a commonly used agent to maintain or re-open the ductus arteriosus in certain congenital heart defects. Which of the following sites is responsible for approximately 80% of the metabolism of alprostadil?

    A. Kidneys
    B. Liver
    C. Lungs
    D. Red blood cell

148. What is an expected heart rate for a healthy full term neonate?

    A. 60 beats/minute
    B. 90 beats/minute
    C. 160 beats/minute
    D. 220 beats/minute

149. In a healthy term neonate you can expect the following for a single dose of rocuronium with regards to: onset, clearance, and potency?

    A. Decreased, decreased, increased
    B. Decreased, increased, increased
    C. Increased, decreased, increased
    D. Increased, increased, decreased

150. Which of the following is a name/description frequently used to describe the murmur associated with patent ductus arteriosus?

    A. Austin Flint
    B. "Machine like"
    C. "Mill-wheel"
    D. Still's

151. The highest oxygen saturation you can expect in fetal circulation is approximately 70%. Which of the following anatomical structures correlates with this saturation?

    A. Ductus arteriosus
    B. Aorta
    C. Umbilical artery
    D. Umbilical vein

152. All of the following are compensatory mechanisms for low oxygen partial pressure in the fetus, except:

    A. Decreased oxygen binding
    B. Hemoglobin F
    C. Increased cardiac output
    D. Increased hematocrit

153. Which of the following statements is most accurate when comparing morbidity and mortality rates for anesthesia in pediatric and adult patients?

    A. Adult patients and pediatric patients have identical risk for morbidity and mortality
    B. Adult patients have increased risk for morbidity and mortality
    C. Pediatric patients have increased risk for morbidity and mortality
    D. This data has not been documented

154. The p50 of hemoglobin F is approximately?

    A. 19 mmHg
    B. 26 mmHg
    C. 30 mmHg
    D. 50 mmHg

155. Neonates are known to have increased cardiovascular risks for local anesthetic toxicity. Which of the following is the most likely explanation for this increased risk?

    A. Decreased protein concentration
    B. Decreased weight
    C. Increased blood-brain barrier penetration
    D. Increased cardiac output

156. Normal intracranial pressure for neonate is:

    A. 0 – 2 mmHg
    B. 2 – 6 mmHg
    C. 7 – 15 mmHg
    D. > 15 mmHg

157. Which of the following patients has the highest cerebral blood flow on an mL/100g/minute basis?

    A. 27-week-gestation newborn
    B. 1-month-old
    C. 2-year-old
    D. 15 year-old

Questions #158- 160 Matching: Properties of Local Anesthetics

158. _____ Onset   A. Lipid solubility

159. _____ Duration   B. pKa

160. _____ Potency   C. Protein binding

161. Hemodilution is routinely utilized during pediatric and adult cardiopulmonary bypass to improve which of the following?

    A. End tidal carbon dioxide
    B. Oxygen saturation
    C. Perfusion
    D. Temperature

162. You are planning an inhalation mask induction. In which of the following patients do you anticipate marked bradycardia during your induction?

    A. 3-year-old otherwise healthy patient
    B. 3-year-old with attention deficit disorder
    C. 3-year-old with Down syndrome
    D. 3-year-old with latex allergy

163. Both fetal and adult neuromuscular junctions have five subunits. Which of the following subunits is only found in the fetal neuromuscular junction?

    A. Alpha subunit
    B. Beta subunit
    C. Epsilon subunit
    D. Gamma subunit

164. Etomidate is only FDA (Federal Drug Agency) approved for children greater than what age?

   A. 1 month old
   B. 6 months old
   C. 1 year old
   D. 10 years old

165. The potency of rocuronium should be expected to be greatest in which of the following patients?

   A. 2 months old
   B. 2 years old
   C. 10 years old
   D. 14 years old

166. Which of the following parameters is reduced in neonates?

   A. Cardiac output
   B. Oxygen consumption
   C. Respiratory rate
   D. Tissue: gas solubility

167. Which of the following ages typically correlates to the developmental milestone of separation anxiety in otherwise healthy infants?

   A. 4 – 6 months
   B. 6 – 12 months
   C. 12 – 18 months
   D. Separation anxiety is considered abnormal development

168. You are called to assist with an emergency C-section delivery for late decelerations with contractions. The amniotic fluid is noted to be stained with meconium. The infant is delivered and has a 1-minute APGAR of 2. After stimulating and warming, what is the best next step in management of this child?

   A. Bag mask ventilate to improve oxygen saturations
   B. Bulb suction the nares and oropharynx; apply CPAP
   C. Intubate and suction meconium contents from lungs
   D. Place oral-gastric tube and suction contents

Questions #169-174 Matching: Pharmacology

169. _____ Nitroglycerine

170. _____ Sodium nitroprusside

171. _____ Phentolamine

172. _____ Hydralazine

173. _____ Prostaglandin E1

174. _____ Esmolol

   A. Dilates both arterial and venous capacitance vessels. Can cause reflex tachycardia in addition to cyanide toxicity.
   B. Direct acting smooth muscle dilator with a long duration of action. Can cause lupus like syndrome, drug fever, and thrombocytopenia
   C. Direct smooth muscle relaxation, can cause apnea in neonates.
   D. Predominately dilates venous capacitance vessels by smooth muscle relaxation.
   E. Selective alpha receptor blocker, greatest effect on arterial vessels.
   F. Short acting beta blocker (beta 1 selective). Rapid onset/offset.

175. At what site should a pulse oximetry probe be placed in order to give the shortest delay in response to desaturation?

   A. Ear
   B. Finger
   C. Head
   D. Toe

176. All of the following medications can be given via the endotracheal route in a 1 year old, except?

   A. Atropine
   B. Vasopressin
   C. Epinephrine
   D. Lidocaine

177. You are asked to provide anesthesia for an 8-year-old child scheduled for an MRI. The patient's medical history is significant for an intracranial mass. All of the following are known to decrease intracranial pressure (ICP) except:

   A. Hyperventilation
   B. Sevoflurane
   C. Mannitol
   D. Steroids

Questions #178-182 Matching: Respiratory Volumes

178. _____ Dead space (V_D)

179. _____ Functional residual capacity (FRC)

180. _____ Tidal volume (TV)

181. _____ Total lung capacity (TLC) adult

182. _____ Total lung capacity (TLC) infant

   A. 2.5 ml/kg
   B. 7 ml/kg
   C. 30 ml/kg
   D. 63 ml/kg
   E. 82 ml/kg

183. It is well known that massive blood transfusion can result in hypocalcemia. Which of the following ECG changes indicates hypocalcemia?

   A. J waves
   B. Peaked T waves
   C. Prolonged QT interval
   D. U waves

Chapter 13 Answers with Explanations

#1 Answer: B) *0.01 mg/kg, or 10mcg/kg*

Asystole or PEA algorithm includes: call for help, turn off all anesthetic gases, 100% O2, place patient on backboard, start chest compressions (100/min +8 breaths/min), maximize $ETCO_2$ >10 mmHg, allow full recoil of chest, do not stop compressions for pulse check, epinephrine 10 mcg/kg every 3-5 min, check pulse every 2 minutes (switch chest compressor at this time) call for ECMO if no return of spontaneous circulation after 6 minutes of CPR. *(American Heart Association 2010 recommendations)*

#2 Answer: A) *Give intra-muscular succinylcholine*

Laryngospasm is a true airway emergency. It is a clinical event seen commonly in pediatric anesthesia. The patient is attempting to move air (the diaphragm is working) but the vocal cords are closed, preventing air movement in and out of the lungs. The **rate limiting step clinically is recognition** that the patient is in laryngospasm. Barash provides a flow chart algorithm, which lists step-by-step interventions: Call for help, give 100% oxygen, attempt airway maneuver: oral airway, double jaw thrust, positive pressure breath. If these measures are unsuccessful, give succinylcholine IV or intramuscular (if no IV).

#3 Answer: A) *Decreased blood:gas solubility*

The rate of mask induction is determined predominately by four factors: solubility of agent, rate of increase of inspired concentration, maximal inspired concentration, and respirations. Inspired concentration determines the rise of alveolar concentration. Alveolar concentration and solubility determines blood concentration which determines brain concentration. Less soluble agents (nitrous, sevoflurane, desflurane) are taken up by the blood at a decreased rate, which increases alveolar concentration. This effect is further enhanced in the pediatric population where blood solubility is further decreased. Please remember that minimum alveolar concentration is roughly the same for adults as for children, though MAC does decrease slightly per decade. An increased cardiac output will actually delay induction; the greater the blood flow through the lungs the greater the uptake of gases, the slower the rise of alveolar gas concentration. Minute ventilation is dramatically increased in infants, and increases onset.

#4 Answer: D) *Ventricular septal defect*

Some of the more common congenital cardiac defects include: ventricular septal defect 16%, transposition of the great arteries 10%, tetralogy of Fallot 9%, coarctation of aorta 8%, hypoplastic left heart 7.9%, atrial septal defect 3%. *(Smiths, 7th edition, pg. 577)*

#5 Answer: D) *Thrombocytopenia*

NEC can be a life-threatening emergency. While almost exclusively found in premature infants, it is possible for a term infant to develop NEC. Pathophysiology is not completely understood, but it is believe to be related to ischemia of the bowel. There are many signs and symptoms associated with NEC: feeding intolerance, respiratory compromise, hypovolemia, hypotension, abdominal distension, apnea, thrombocytopenia leading to coagulopathy, and organ failure. A perforated bowel will typically result in elevated lactic acid, and possible hemodynamic instability. In a sick neonate, hypoglycemia is far more common than hyperglycemia; anemia is also very likely to be present. Hallmarks of treatment include: antibiotics, parental nutrition, bowel rest (NPO), vasopressors for hemodynamic instability, and surgical intervention for bowel perforation. *(Cote, 4th edition, pg. 742)*

#6 Answer: D) *Succinylcholine*

Of the drugs listed, only succinylcholine has a black box warning. **Risk of cardiac arrests from hyperkalemic rhabdomyolysis** is listed in the warning. The warning states that succinylcholine should be reserved in pediatrics for emergency airways only; examples include: RSI, full stomach, and airway emergencies (laryngospasm). The black box warning came into effect after several cases of pediatric death following use of succinylcholine. Treatment for cardiac arrest following succinylcholine should follow PALS algorithm for cardiac arrest, in addition to treatment for hyperkalemia: IV calcium, bicarbonate, glucose + insulin and hyperventilation. *(fda.gov)*

#7 Answer: A) *Duchene Muscular dystrophy*

Several pediatric deaths occurred in the 1980s in patients with undiagnosed Duchenne muscular dystrophy following the use of succinylcholine. It is well documented that the release of potassium following muscle contractions induced by succinylcholine will cause life-threatening hyperkalemia is these patients.
Pharmacology review: succinylcholine is a rapid acting, **depolarizing** neuromuscular relaxant. As succinylcholine binds the neuromuscular nicotinic receptors, ionic channels open- K^+ out, Na^+ in. Severe hyperkalemia can occur after a single dose in the following conditions: lower motor neuron (tetanus), upper motor neuron (paraplegia, spinal cord injuries), burns >8% BSA, neuromuscular diseases: Duchenne, Beckers MD, crush injuries. Duchenne muscular dystrophy is a disease that affects multiple organs; specifically these patients have abnormal muscle formation, and have an upregulation of immature ACh receptors. Immature or fetal receptors have many differences from adult receptors; specifically they remain open 2 – 10-fold longer, which in turns provides longer duration of potassium efflux. Sinus bradycardia is a known risk of succinylcholine; typically you will encounter this after a second dose/bolus, although it can happen with first dose. *(Smith's 7th ed, pg. 214, Cote 4th ed, pg. 128)*

#8 Answer: B) *Increased*

> Incidence considered 1:15,000 in pediatric vs 1:50,000 in adults. The explanation for the increased incidence in pediatrics is not well understood.

#9 Answer: D) *X-linked recessive - Duchenne muscular dystrophy (males only)*
   A) *Autosomal dominant - Malignant hyperthermia*
   D) *X-linked recessive - Hemophilia A (males only)*
   B) *Autosomal recessive - Cystic fibrosis*

> Malignant hyperthermia is considered autosomal dominant with incomplete penetrance. Incomplete penetrance means that not as many inherit the disease as would be predicted based on AD inheritance pattern. In autosomal dominant inheritance, one parent needs to carry the gene mutation, offspring who inherit the copy of the gene mutation will have the disease.

#10 Answer: A) *Chromosome #19*

> Multiple chromosomes are being studied in regards to MH, and more than 160 mutations have been identified in the ryanodine RYRI receptor, however chromosome #19 is considered the location of the RYRI gene. *(Cote 4th ed, pg. 856)*

#11 Answer: B) *Increased ETCO$_2$*

> All of the above are likely clinical signs of malignant hyperthermia. Of the choices listed, increased ETCO$_2$ would be the first sign. In fact increased ETCO$_2$ is responsible for the other signs/symptoms listed. Recall that MH is a hypermetabolic state, increased oxygen consumption with increased CO$_2$ production. This is in addition to abnormal muscle spasm/contracture. An arterial gas would be expected to show a mixed respiratory/metabolic acidosis (high PaCO$_2$, low HCO$_3$).

#12 Answer: C) *Postpone MRI until patient is beyond one month of age*

> In an otherwise completely healthy full term neonate, there is no reason to anesthetize the patient for an elective procedure than can reasonably wait several weeks. Based on an algorithm presented in Cote, full-term neonates less than 30 days old the following considerations should be implemented: First case of the day, consider regional block if applicable, extended PACU stay, admit to monitored bed overnight. If the otherwise healthy infant is greater than 30 days old, the following considerations are recommended: schedule as first case of the day, consider regional block, extended PACU stay, discharge home only if completely uneventful recovery, adequate pain control and fluid intake. *(Cote 4th edition, pg. 67, Gregory 4th ed, pg 361)*

#13 Answer: C) *L3*

The neonatal spinal cord tip is typically more caudad (lower) in the spinal canal than that of an adult. A neonate's cord will generally extend all the way down to L3. As one grows the cord tip moves cephalad (higher) reaching an adult level of L1 – L2 by the age of one year old. *(Cote 4th ed, pg. 875)*

#14 Answer: D) *Withdraw needle, abort procedure*

Spiked T waves are considered a positive test dose, indicating likely intravascular injection of local anesthetic. The most prudent course of action is to withdraw the needle, and abort the procedure. Negative aspiration does not completely ensure that the needle is not intravascular or intrathecal. Repeating a test dose without repositioning the needle would be a mistake. Consider the following a positive test does after injection of local anesthetic: T wave changes, HR increases greater than 10 beats/minute, or systolic blood pressure increase greater than 10%. While the patient should continue to be monitored for systemic toxicity, no further pharmacological interventions are indicated based on a positive test dose in isolation. *(Cote 4th ed, pg. 872)*

#15 Answer: D) *The same*

FRC is approximately 30 ml/kg in both adults and neonates. In fact several of the respiratory volumes are considered the same on an ml/kg basis, including tidal volumes (6-8ml/kg), as well as dead space (2 – 3ml/kg). Please keep in mind that absolute respiratory volumes are clearly less in a neonate. It is important to point out that alveolar ventilation of a neonate is significantly INCREASED vs an adult. Remember the formula for alveolar ventilation $V_A = (V_T - V_D) \times RR$. Alveolar ventilation is INCREASED in neonates secondary to increased respiratory rates. Increased alveolar ventilation in neonates is necessary secondary to the INCREASED O_2 consumption. A neonate's O_2 consumption is approximately 6 – 8 ml/kg/min vs an adult's which is 3 – 4 ml/kg/min.
* V_A = alveolar ventilation, V_T = Tidal volume, V_D = Dead space volume.

#16 Answer: D) *Sickle cell hemoglobin*

Fetal Hb F has a P_{50} of approximately 19 mmHg, this is a left shift from the adult Hb A P_{50} of 26 mmHg. Decreased 2,3-DPG, alkalosis, hypothermia as well as methemoglobin are all considered classic examples of a left-shift on the oxygen hemoglobin curve. A left-shift indicates that the hemoglobin molecule has an **INCREASED** affinity to oxygen (tighter bond), less O_2 partial pressure is needed to have 50% of the hemoglobin saturated. Sickle cell anemia on the other hand has a P_{50}=31mmHg, the sickle hemoglobin Hb SS has a **DECREASED** affinity for the oxygen, thus an increased partial pressure of oxygen is required to achieve a 50% saturation of the hemoglobin. *(Morgan & Mikhail's 5th ed, pg 1177)*

#17 Answer: A) *Increased diastolic pressure*

The ductus arteriosus remains patent is approximately 1:2,500 live births. At birth the normal physiologic changes include a rise in SVR and a decrease in PRV (secondary to oxygen). If the ductus remains open, what was a right to left shunt in-utero will now become a left to right shunt, as ratio of SVR > PVR. A PDA causes diastolic runoff, with a widened pulse pressure (increased difference between systolic and diastolic pressure), this runoff (aortic blood meant for systemic circulation, flowing through ductus to lungs) lowers the diastolic pressures. Once the shunt has been eliminated you should see a rise in the diastolic pressure, it is usually immediate and is a noticeable change on your arterial pressure line.

#18 Answer: D) *Sacrococcygeal ligament*

The sacrococcygeal ligament lies directly over the sacral hiatus; this is the correct location for needle insertion while performing a caudal.

#19 Answer: C) *Order an MRI scan*

Epidural abscess is considered a potential clinical emergency. The reported incidence is 1:500,000. Most cases involve a catheter. Based on the above description and patient's history, you should have a high index of suspicion for an epidural abscess. Additional signs and symptoms of an epidural abscess include: increased SED rate, left-shift white blood cell count, back pain, paraplegia, sensory loss, urinary/ fecal retention, local tenderness. MRI is the recommended diagnostic test, and should be obtained as soon as possible. Blood cultures, as well as expressed pus should be sent to determine exact organism. Additional labs to order also include a CBC and SED rate. Consult Neurosurgery in addition to Infectious Disease. An epidural abscess can result in sepsis and paraplegia if not addressed in a timely fashion. Broad-based antibiotics should be initiated awaiting results of cultures. *(COTE 4th ed, pg. 883, Morgan & Mikhail 5th ed, pg. 971)*

#20 Answer: C) *Mandibular hypoplasia, macrostomia, cleft palate*

Treacher Collins syndrome patients present with mandibular hypoplasia, cleft palate, macrostomia, Hypoplastic zygomatic arches, possible cardiac defects and renal anomalies. These patients are considered to have a **difficult airway** until proven otherwise. *(Cote 4th ed, pg. 708)*

#21 Answer: D) *Micrognathia, glossoptosis, respiratory distress*

Pierre Robin syndrome consists of micrognathia, glossoptosis, and respiratory distress in the first 24 hours (+/- cleft palate). They are considered a **difficult airway**. Pierre Robin syndrome patients frequently come to the OR in the first two months of life for mandibular distraction, which usually alleviates the difficult airway. Even without the surgical intervention, the airway does improve with age. *(Cote 4th ed, pg. 709)*

#22 Answer: B) *Macroglossia, gigantism, hypoglycemia*

Beckwith-Wiedemann syndrome consists of macroglossia, gigantism, organomegaly, possible omphalocele as well as hypoglycemia. They commonly have congenital heart defects as well. Expect macroglossia; they may or may not be a difficult airway. *(Cote pg. 274)*

#23 Answer: A) *Unilateral hemifacial hypoplasia, absent ear*

Goldenhar syndrome consists of unilateral hemifacial hypoplasia, with an absent ear. These patients are considered a **difficult airway**. They come to the operating for serial plastics procedures. *(Cote 4th ed, pg. 274)*

#24 Answer: B) *Non-Hodgkin lymphoma, see #28 explanation*

#25 Answer: B) *An ECHO, see #28 explanation*

#26 Answer: D) *Placing chest tube with local anesthetic, see #28 explanation*

#27 Answer: C) *Place patient in lateral decubitus position, see #28 explanation*

#28 Answer: D) *Tracheal compression >50% on CT scan*

Mediastinal mass differential diagnosis: lymphoma (#1), Hodgkin, thymoma, and teratoma. Studies/ workup should include: CT scan evaluate airway, size location of mass, chest X-ray, ECHO, PFTs, MRI (not ideal if patient cannot lay flat due to respiratory compromise), CBC, coagulation profile, type and cross +/-. If patient has respiratory compromise with supine position, general anesthesia is considered contraindicated; recommend biopsy under local anesthesia. If patient is not compromised and anesthesia can be tolerated, it is recommended to leave the patient spontaneously breathing, as muscle relaxation can result in complete airway collapse if the mass crushes the airway when gravity takes over as the natural resting muscle tension that the chest cavity provides is removed. If the airway becomes compromised at any time during procedure turning the patient in a lateral decubitus or even prone position may release the mass effect on the trachea/airway/heart. Bad prognostic indicators with high likelihood of intra-op and post-op respiratory compromise include: +respiratory compromise with supine position, restrictive/obstructive dysfunction on PFTs, >50% tracheal compression from mass on CT.

#29 Answer: B) *Choanal atresia*

VACTERL: V= vertebral anomalies, A = anal atresia (colon not affected), C = cardiac, TE = tracheoesophageal fistula, R = renal anomalies, L = limb anomalies (radial)

#30 Answer: C) *Prostaglandin E1*

Hypercarbia, acidosis, hypoxia, upper respiratory infections, crying (stress), as well as hypothermia can INCREASE pulmonary vascular resistance. Prostaglandin F2 (dinoprost), provides smooth muscle contraction and is used for postpartum hemorrhage. Prostaglandin E1 (alprostadil) provides smooth muscle relaxation, 80% is metabolized by the lungs, adverse drug reactions include: apnea, fever, hypotension, flushing, bradycardia and cardiac arrest.

#31 Answer: D) *Lidocaine and prilocaine*

EMLA cream is a mixture of lidocaine and prilocaine - both amides. It is commonly used as a topical agent to provide analgesia for intravenous needle sticks. EMLA generally requires 20 – 30 minutes for good topicalization. Side effects and warnings: prilocaine can cause methemoglobin, other concerns: skin blanching, erythema, itching. Extreme caution should be used if patients are already receiving methemoglobinemia inducing medications: phenobarbital, dapsone, sulfa drugs. *(Cote 4th edition, p 869)*

#32 Answer: A) *2-week-old male*

Cardiopulmonary pump flow rates are determined by metabolic demand. The smaller the child, the higher the metabolic demand. Recommended flow rates for cardiopulmonary bypass, are weight based. *(Lake, 4th ed, p 241)*

#33 Answer: C) *Hypocarbia*

Moyamoya is a disease of the intracranial vessels, predominately the internal carotid. Radiographically referred to as "puff of smoke", associated with Down syndrome and Neurofibromatosis type 1. Aneurysms are possible, and TIAs are common. The TIAs are thought to be associated with hyperventilation resulting in hypocarbia. Recall hypocarbia → cerebral vasoconstriction → decreased blood flow → possible stroke. Even mild hyperventilation should be avoided on the ventilator. Post operatively, be aware of a crying patient (increased RR, increased TV) as this can result in stroke.

#34 Answer: D) *Red blood cell*

Red blood cells are the site of metabolism for nitric oxide.

$$Red\ blood\ cell + iNO \rightarrow nitrate + methemoglobin$$

Beware of increasing metHb levels that may require monitoring.
Pulmonary hypertension creates a V/Q mismatch two mechanisms possible: vasoconstriction decreases pulmonary blood flow and shunting right to left resulting in hypoxia. iNO produces pulmonary vasodilation.

#35 Answer: C) *18%*

The head of a neonate comprises approximately 18% of its body surface area, compared with an adult in which the head comprises 9% of total body surface area. The head of a neonate can be a large source for heat loss in the operating room. Thin bones of the skull, open fontanelles, decreased hair (insulation), thin skin all increase mechanisms for heat loss. Care should always be taken to cover the infants head with plastic or a blanket. *(Cote, 4th ed, p 560)*

#36 Answer: B) *Crying*

All of the choices except crying are considered interventions for a hypercyanotic spell or "tet spell". The tet spell results in increased right-to-left shunting (unoxygenated blood) via the VSD, possibly secondary to infundibular muscle spasm at the level of the right ventricular out flow tract. This shunting of blood results in hypoxia, and cyanosis. Crying increases pulmonary vascular resistance (PVR), increasing PVR results in increased right-to-left shunting. Remember when opportunity exists i.e. communication (VSD) between right and left heart, pulmonary vascular resistance and systemic vascular resistance will determine which direction the blood flows. It will take the path of least resistance, i.e. high to low pressure.

Treatment goals for tet spells:
- Fluids - reverse hypovolemia
- Increase depth of anesthesia
- Fentanyl - slow heart rate, decrease catecholamines
- Increase SVR - with phenylephrine
- 100% oxygen

(Lake 4th ed, p 345- 346, 349)

#37 Answer: D) *β-sympathetic fibers*

Multiple nerve fibers are involved in thermal regulation. Brown fat is predominately innervated by β-sympathetic fibers. A-delta fibers are responsible for afferent impulses (from periphery to central) for cold sensitive receptors; C-fibers transmit hot impulses from peripheral receptors. A-gamma fibers are motor fibers. *(Cote 4th ed, p 562)*

38 Answer: B) *60 mg*

Divide total heparin dose by 100. 1 mg protamine is given for every 100 units of heparin, or protamine at a dose of 4 mg/kg. Heparin's dosage is weight-based, though the exact amount units/kg varies from institution to institution, can range from 200 – 400 units/kg. Heparin and protamine create a neutralization reaction, thus reversing the effects of heparin.

#39 Answer: D) *Potassium*

Neonates have decreased GFR and a decreased ability to concentrate their urine, thus normal serum potassium for a neonate 0 – 1 month old can range from 4 – 6.0 mEq/L. A neonate would be far more prone to hypoglycemia than hyperglycemia. Production of urea is decreased and an elevated BUN in an infant represents renal failure. Bicarbonate levels are also reduced in neonates, normally 22 mEq/L vs adult 24 mEq/L. (*Cote 4th ed, p 570*)

#40 Answer: A) *Anaphylaxis*

Anaphylaxis classic presenting signs/symptoms: bronchospasm (increased peak airway pressures, desaturation), hypotension, flushing.

#41 Answer: B) *Epinephrine*

The question describes a classic presentation of anaphylaxis. Anaphylaxis usually presents within seconds of the triggering agent, in this case, clindamycin. Muscle relaxants are the number one offender in the OR, antibiotics are number two. Bronchospasm is almost immediate with increased peak airway pressures, decreased tidal volumes, and decreased saturation. Bronchospasm can present as wheezing, however if severe enough you can have diminished breath sounds, and even no breath sounds are actually possible. Hypotension will ensue but is generally after the onset of pulmonary reaction. Classic anaphylaxis triad: bronchospasm, hypotension, flushing. Treatment is supportive: stop offending agent, 100% oxygen, open intravenous fluids, EPINEPHRINE, steroid, and diphenhydramine (Benadryl). If no intervention, it can result in cardiovascular collapse and death.
Remember: epinephrine at low dose = β effects= bronchodilation
             epinephrine at high/code dose = α effects= vasoconstriction

#42 Answer: D) *Ventricular septal defect*

Ductal-dependent lesions = hearts that cannot supply systemic or pulmonary perfusion. Generally these are congenital cardiac lesions that result in an absent or grossly impaired right or left side of the heart, or severe anomalies of the aorta or pulmonary artery. There are multiple congenital cardiac lesions that must depend on a patent, or open ductus arteriosus (pulmonary artery to aorta connection) to provide either systemic or pulmonary blood flow. Some of these lesions include: hypoplastic left heart, transposition of the great arteries, pulmonary atresia, tricuspid atresia, and critical aortic stenosis.

#43 Answer: A) *Aluminum*

Ferromagnetic metals or those that contain **lead** are considered dangerous in an MRI suite. Ferromagnetic metals will react with the powerful magnetic field created by the MRI. The following are considered non-ferrous metals: aluminum, copper, lead, nickel, tin, titanium, and zinc. Of note gold, silver, and platinum are also non-ferrous. Always check your pockets before entering the MRI suite. Deaths have occurred in the MRI suite from metal-magnet attraction. Metal becomes a missile in MRI suite.

#44 Answer: A) *Desflurane*

    Percentage metabolized:
    Halothane 20% > sevoflurane 5% > isoflurane 0.2% > **desflurane <0.01%**

#45 Answer: B) *4 hours*

    2,4,6,8 who do we appreciate? Parents who follow the NPO guidelines!
- 2 hrs - Clears
- 4 hrs - Breast milk
- 6 hrs - Formula, G-tube feed, cow's milk, light meal
- 8 hrs - Heavy meal (fats/protein) – e.g. McDonald's happy meal

#46 Answer: D) *Atrial septal defect*

    Cyanosis is typically seen in the following congenital cardiac lesions: Single ventricles (right or left sided), right-to-left shunts (tetralogy of Fallot), truncus arteriosus, tricuspid atresia, pulmonary atresia, and transposition of great vessels. Ebstein anomaly with mixing lesions AV canal may or may not have cyanosis. Cyanosis is also present in pulmonary hypertension from any etiology: cardiac, pulmonary (RSV), persistent pulmonary hypertension of newborn. Atrial and ventricular septal defects are typically acyanotic. *(Cote, 4th ed, p 34)*

#47 Answer: D) *Thumbprint sign*

    Epiglottitis is generally considered an airway emergency due to the possibility of complete airway obstruction secondary to edema of the epiglottis, subglottic as well as supraglottic tissue. The recognizable" thumb print" on x-ray is the swollen epiglottis, best seen on a lateral head/ neck film.
    Haemophilus influenzae type B has been virtually eradicated with immunization (be alert for unvaccinated children), however Group A β-hemolytic Strep may cause same infectious disease process. If the airway must be secured for protection, ENT must be present, and the procedure should commence in the OR, as opposed to the emergency room.
(Cote 4th ed, p 676)

#48 Answer: B) *Cranial nerve V*

    The oculocardiac reflex, or the "five and dime reflex" (which refers to its cranial nerves) is responsible for the bradycardia in this scenario. Cranial Nerve V - the trigeminal nerve, specifically the ophthalmic division (V_1) - is the afferent limb and Cranial Nerve X, the vagus nerve, is the efferent limb. This reflex is in response to ocular muscle retraction or pressure on the globe. In general, it is not considered preventable, however treatment includes: notify the surgeon to release the tension. Possible medication intervention is atropine if necessary. In most cases once the surgeon takes off the retractor, the heart rate increases and returns quickly to baseline.

#49 Answer: A) *Cricothyroid muscle*

The left recurrent laryngeal nerve is located posterior to the aortic arch and wraps around the aorta at the junction of the ductus arteriosus (the site of surgery in this question) and therefore is susceptible to injury during a PDA ligation. The left recurrent laryngeal nerve (left RLN) is a branch of the cranial nerve X (Vagus). Injury to the RLN nerve can result in paralysis of the one muscle that opens (abduction) the vocals cords: the posterior cricoarytenoid muscle; injury to the RLN will leave the cord at the midline position or closed, resulting in hoarseness and may impair respiration. RLN also innervates the lateral cricoarytenoid muscle, as well as the thyroarytenoid muscle. The cricothyroid muscle is innervated by the Superior Laryngeal Nerve, also a branch of the Vagus.

#50 Answer: B) *Postpone case for 6 hours, following NPO guidelines*

NPO guidelines for formula recommend 6 hours. Pyloric stenosis is NOT a surgical emergency. It is however considered a full stomach regardless of NPO status; this patient is considered high risk for aspiration. No matter how long you wait after last PO intake there will be milk in the stomach. If you induce this patient who has just been fed, there is a high likelihood of aspiration. For pyloric stenosis patients, it is standard of care to wait for NPO guidelines to be satisfied. (*ASA Practice Guidelines for Perioperative Fasting, 2011*)

#51 Answer: A) *True*

Incidence: males > female (*Cote 4th ed, p. 761*)

#52 Answer: D) *Metabolic alkalosis with hypokalemia and hypochloremia*

Classic lab presentation for an un-resuscitated pyloric stenosis baby
- **Metabolic alkalosis with HYPOkalemia, and HYPOchloremia.**

One way to help remember these parameters...the baby is projectile vomiting
- HCl^- (stomach acid) out with vomiting
- Cl^- out, so chloride should go down (hypochloremia)
- H^+ acid out so the patient should become alkalotic

With alkalosis you will have potassium driven into cells so hypokalemia should ensue. Simply put, it is metabolic because the lungs are not involved.

#53 Answer: B) *Mask induction with N_2O/O_2 and 8% sevoflurane*

An awake intubation can be used if difficult airway suspected in addition to full stomach. Awake intubation maintains the gag reflex as well as spontaneous respirations avoiding inability to ventilate intubate. Rapid sequence induction is the recommended technique for pyloric stenosis, and can be performed with succinylcholine or RSI dose of rocuronium. A mask induction should never be attempted in this patient, who will almost certainly aspirate with an unsecured airway and a full stomach.

#54 Answer: A) *Mitral valve*

>Marfan disease is a result of a mutation in the fibrillin-1 gene; it affects many systems including the heart. Fibrillin is a protein present in connective tissue; connective tissue is present in the following tissue: bone, ligaments, cartilage, and adipose. This disease primarily affects skeletal, ocular and cardiovascular systems. Lesions that are common in Marfan disease are mitral valve prolapsed and mitral insufficiency. Joint laxity, scoliosis, and restrictive lung disease pattern, spontaneous pneumothorax, and recurrent lung infections are possible.

#55 Answer: D) *Increased v waves*

>Increased v waves are prominent and usually noticeable in the CVP tracing correlating a junctional rhythm diagnosis. Junctional rhythms are not tolerated well when the lack of atrial filling (no P, no atrial contraction) result in hypotension. *(Cote 4th ed, p 314-315)*
>*a wave= atrial contraction, c wave= tricuspid bulging, v wave= systolic atrium filling, x descent= atrial relaxation, y descent= ventricular filling

#56 Answer: B) *17.5 mg*

>2.5 mg/kg is the maximum allowable dosage for 0.25% bupivacaine with epinephrine.
>   7 kg × 2.5 mg/kg = 17.5 mg total maximum dose for the caudal in this patient
>Calculations are simple when using the above concentration
>- 1 ml of 0.25% bupivacaine with epinephrine = 2.5 mg of bupivacaine
>- Maximum allowable volume you may use is 1ml/kg
>- This is a pediatric calculation shortcut

#57 Answer: C) *Pulmonary atresia*

>Pulmonary atresia is considered a right-to-left shunt. Inhalation inductions with right-to-left shunts (tetralogy of Fallot) can be prolonged. These shunts have diminished or absent pulmonary blood flow so although the alveoli are receiving the anesthetic gas (ventilation), the blood is not picking up the gas (no exchange). If blood is bypassing the lungs, volatile agent is not reaching the brain. Typically ASDs and VSDs are considered left-to-right shunts. However, it is always possible for a left-to-right shunt to convert to a right-to-left shunt if PVR becomes greater than SVR. Coarctation usually does not result in a shunt, but causes diminished blood flow distal to the coarctation - i.e. the lower extremities; you should have a normal inhalation mask induction. Inhalation mask induction (with volatile agents) is NOT ideal for patients with severe congenital heart defects, and even less ideal for patients with right to left shunts.

#58 Answer: B) *Term infant*

>CSF volume ml/kg is as follows: infant > preterm infant > child > adult. A term infant can have from 14 – 16 ml/kg of CSF compared to an adult with 2 – 3 ml/kg. *(Cote 4th ed, p 876)*

#59 Answer: C) *1.25 mg*

To convert percent (%) concentration to milligram per milliliter (mg/ml) multiple by 10, in other words move the decimal point one place to the right. 1.25 mg is correct.

#60 Answer: B) *V_2 - Maxillary division*

For cleft lip repair a regional nerve block technique may be used. The infraorbital nerve block is recommended for this surgical procedure. There are two branches of the infraorbital nerves, a right and a left branch. These are sensory nerves. They are a branch of trigeminal cranial nerve (CN V)—more specifically—maxillary division V_2. This block is considered ideal for lip repairs, and the vermillion. *(Cote 4th ed, p 886)*

#61 Answer: B) *False*

Males > females for cleft lips

#62 Answer: A) *True*

#63 Answer: B) *Pierre Robin syndrome*

There are many syndromes that have an associated cleft palate and or cleft lip. Of those listed, Pierre Robin has an 80% associated cleft palate/lip, Treacher Collins is 28%, Klippel-Feil is 15 %. Other syndromes that may have cleft palate/lip: hemifacial microsomia, Stickler syndrome, down syndrome, fetal alcohol syndrome. *(Somerville N and Fenlon S. Anaesthesia for cleft lip and palate surgery. Continuing Education in Anaesthesia, Critical Care & Pain, vol 5, number 3, 2005)*

#64 Answer: B) *Methemoglobinemia*

The above scenario describes a case of methemoglobinemia that is unresponsive to supplemental oxygen. The patient's pulse oximetry saturation will typically read 80 – 90%. If you were to draw labs on the above patient, the blood would have a "chocolate brown color." Normal methemoglobin levels are 1 – 3%; >10% is considered a level that requires intervention. Methylene blue is the prescribed treatment. Primary brain tumor patients are routinely prescribed dapsone as prophylaxis for Pneumocystis jiroveci pneumonia. Signs symptoms of methemoglobinemia include cyanotic features, decreasing mentation, and confusion. *(Cote 4th ed, p 192)*

#65 Answer: D) *Dapsone*

Dapsone is the offending agent with a known side effect of methemoglobinemia. Primary brain tumor patients are routinely prescribed dapsone as prophylaxis for Pneumocystis jiroveci pneumonia. Risks factors for developing methemoglobinemia in patients taking dapsone are anemia and advanced age. Approximately 5 – 20% who take dapsone will develop methemoglobinemia.

#66 Answer: D) *All of the above*

All of the syndromes listed – Down, Goldenhar and Pierre Robin – are predisposed to airway obstruction. Almost all craniofacial syndromes are predisposed to airway obstruction, secondary to the physical bone and muscle/tissue structure of the head. Several key features lead to likelihood of airway obstruction: small mouth, large tongue, retrognathia (jaw displaced posteriorly), mandibular hypoplasia, micrognathia (smaller than normal jaw), and large head: body ratio (produces head flexion). Oh and don't forget…narcotics!

Narcotics = 👿, patients with OSA are exquisitely sensitive to effects of narcotics!!!!!

#67 Answer: B) *pH-STAT*

pH STAT = pH neutral at patient's actual temperature, CO_2 is generally added to correct for hypothermic-induced relative hypocarbia. Remember that as the body is cooled, $PaCO_2$ will decrease as carbon dioxide becomes increasingly soluble. This method of blood gas analysis is commonly used in pediatrics; benefit is believed to be increased cerebral perfusion. Recall, hypocarbia induces cerebral vasoconstriction which in turn decreases cerebral perfusion rather effectively. Pay attention to your cerebral oximetry in the pediatric cardiac operating room, and notice the direct effect your end tidal carbon dioxide has on the cerebral oxygen saturation.

#68 Answer: D) *Sevoflurane*

Recall that tetralogy of Fallot is usually a right to left shunt. Unoxygenated blood is shunted from the right ventricle to the left ventricle, via a VSD, bypassing the lungs, therefore the blood is not able to participate in "uptake" of the volatile agent from the alveoli. The agents that are most affected by this phenomenon are the **least soluble** agents: nitrous, desflurane, sevoflurane. You should anticipate no change in onset with intravenous induction (ketamine), or theoretically slightly faster onset, as some of the intravenous drug is carried from venous to arterial circulation, bypassing lungs.

#69 Answer: B) *Duchenne muscular dystrophy*

Duchenne muscular dystrophy has contraindications for succinylcholine (hyperkalemia) and volatile agents (rhabdomyolysis). However, Duchenne is NOT considered MH susceptible. **Diseases considered malignant hyperthermia susceptible are King-Denborough, Core and Multiminicore disease.** (*mhaus.org*)

#70 Answer: D) *Preservative free water*

mhaus.org

#71 Answer: D) *Increased cerebral blood flow*

The mechanisms by which adverse neurological outcomes happen are believed to be different for infants compared to adults. Adult neurological insults are believed to result from thromboembolism, whereas infants are thought to result from ischemia from hypoperfusion. As the carbon dioxide levels go down with hypothermia (drives CO_2 intracellular) during bypass, cerebral vasoconstriction causes decreased cerebral blood flow. Theoretically with pH-Stat you have normal $PaCO_2$ levels that produce minimal change in cerebral vasculature and blood flow. *(Andropoulos 2nd ed, p 111-112)*

#72 Answer: C) *41 weeks*

To calculate post gestational age: add the patients time (weeks) in the womb at delivery (normal gestation =40 weeks) + plus the weeks alive since birth.
    25 weeks gestation in utero, or delivered at 25 weeks
    + 16 weeks alive (4 months old × 4 weeks/month)
    41 weeks post gestational age (PGA)

#73 Answer: C) *Within 6 hours of surgery*

Approximately 75% of tonsillar hemorrhages occur within 6 hours of surgery. Post-op day seven is the second most common time for possible bleed; day #7 is usually the time when the eschar falls off of the wound. The hemorrhage can be severe (internal carotid artery), and may require surgery to control the bleeding. *(Cote 4th ed, p 670)*

#74 Answer: D) *Rapid sequence induction*

A bleeding tonsil is considered an emergency; it is also a full stomach regardless of NPO status, and therefore is high risk for aspiration. A rapid sequence induction is standard of care for this procedure. Prior to the operating room, a CBC should be checked and a type and cross ordered. Pay attention to vital signs (tachycardia and hypotension are bad indicators of significant blood loss). Other considerations include preparation with two suction canisters, succinylcholine or a rapid sequence dose of rocuronium, stylet endotracheal tube, and emergency medications ready - i.e. epinephrine, succinylcholine, atropine, and blood.

#75 Answer: B) *Ketamine*

Based on the patient's vital signs and labs presented, this patient is in critical condition. Perforated bowl? Think septic shock. The procedure is an emergency and delaying the case may result in death. Proceeding with the case, is also likely to be fraught with danger. Of the options, ketamine would most likely be the best choice. Keep in mind there really is no ideal drug for this scenario. Inducing anesthesia in a critically ill patient can result in immediate cardiovascular collapse. Sevoflurane is not an option for induction, and it is possible that the patient will not tolerate the volatile anesthetic after induction. This patient requires a true rapid sequence induction; aspiration risk is high so an inhalation mask induction should be avoided. In this scenario, propofol will likely cause an even greater decrease of SVR and result in profound hypotension. It is possible that even ketamine could result in cardiac/systemic compromise. Etomidate is another option, and least likely to compound hemodynamic instability. There really is no great answer! Have epinephrine and blood ready!!!

#76 Answer: B) *Pulmonary artery blood pressure 2X systemic blood flow*

Definition: Qp:Qs , Qp = pulmonary blood flow, Qs = systemic blood flow.
Normal physiology in an adult heart Qp:Qs should be 1:1, same volume of blood goes to the pulmonic circulation (lungs) as to the systemic circulation (body). With series circulation, blood in the right heart travels to lungs (Qp), left heart blood travels to body (Qs). In certain cardiac lesions, there are communications between the right and left side of the heart creating shunts, these can be right-to-left (cyanotic) or left-to-right (acyanotic, pulmonary over perfusion). In the above scenario, the shunt shows two times the perfusion of the lungs compared to systemic circulation. It is highly likely in this scenario, that the mean pulmonary artery pressure is elevated, and also likely the right atrium and ventricle may be enlarged or with elevated pressures. Strictly based on the question, answer B is correct.

#77 Answer: B) *Maintain spontaneous ventilation*

Airway foreign body is considered an emergency. Airway compromise and obstruction is a possibility which can result in hypoxia and death. A peanut requires emergent retrieval. Morbidity and mortality are twofold: mechanical obstruction from the object and the local response to the peanut which causes an inflammatory response resulting in edema. Maintaining spontaneous ventilation is ideal; you do not want to take away the patient's ability to ventilate as you may run into a situation where by you cannot ventilate this patient. The fear in muscle relaxation, or inhibiting their respiratory drive is an inability to ventilate; if the foreign object obstructs the trachea. An equally important goal is to keep the patient calm for the same reason. An intravenous line is ideal; however it is perfectly acceptable to perform a mask inhalation induction, as spontaneous ventilation is preserved. Please do not induce this patient without the ENT surgeon in the room, their skill and ability with the rigid bronchoscope could be lifesaving. Another maneuver commonly employed if the object completely obstructs trachea is to push object down into right or left mainstem, allowing you to at least ventilate a single lung as opposed to no lungs.

#78 Answer: A) *5*

#79 Answer: D) *Omphalocele*

    Beckwith-Wiedemann syndrome is significant for the following: visceromegaly (enlarged internal organs), hypoglycemia, neonatal polycythemia, +/- mental delay, omphalocele, and possible congenital heart defects. Difficult intubation is listed in the textbooks, most likely secondary to macroglossia. *(Cote 4th ed, p 274)*

#80 Answer: A) *Cystic Fibrosis*

    Cystic Fibrosis (CF) is autosomal recessive, occurring in 1:2000 caucasian live births. Chromosome #7. Electrolyte transport disturbance in epithelial cells causes thick / viscous secretions: affects sweat ducts, airway, pancreatic duct, **intestines**, and vas deferens. Lung disease is primary site of morbidity and cause for mortality. Type 1 diabetes is a common result of pancreatic insufficiency. Nasal polypectomy is the most common reason for presentation of CF patients in pediatric operating rooms. 10 – 15% of infants present with meconium ileus, must r/o CF. Treatment is supportive care for chronic lung infections and nutritional supplementation. Consider lung transplant. *(Cote 4th ed, p 233)*

#81 Answer: A) *<1 year old*

    Less than one year old is the greatest predictor of mortality from child abuse. *www.cdc.gov/violenceprevention/pdf/childmaltreatment-facts-at-a-glance.pdf*

#82 Answer: C) *Chest compressions*

    With HR less than 60, chest compressions should be initiated. Bradycardia secondary to hypoxia, in this case as a result of complete laryngospasm, should be treated with epinephrine. Epinephrine is indicated; however, if you do not initiate chest compressions, the epinephrine given in a peripheral IV may not make it to central circulation or will certainly have a very slow transit time. So in order: **Anesthesia STAT** (get help fast), Succinylcholine, 100% O_2, initiate chest compressions, epi, follow PALS algorithm for bradycardia.
You will NEVER be faulted for calling for help, it shows good judgment, and that you placed the patient's well-being as your priority.

#83 Answer: C) *12 hours*

> The minimum time after a witnessed apneic event to hold and monitor a patient would be 12 hours. Most pediatric hospitals have written policies on admitting ex-premature infants less than 55 – 60 post-gestational age for a period of 24 hours. Postoperative observation times were provided by Cote's highly cited article: *Cote, CJ.1995. Postoperative apnea in former preterm infants after inguinal herniorrhaphy. A combined analysis. Anesthesiology 82 (4), p 809-22*

#84 Answer: C) Na^+ *135, K^+ 2.4, Cl^- 73, CO_2 50*

> The scenario is a classic description of pyloric stenosis. Recall this is a medical emergency. These patients arrive in the emergency room with varying degrees of dehydration secondary to vomiting. They will have metabolic derangements, specifically metabolic alkalosis with: hypokalemia, hypochloremia, hyponatremia, and elevated bicarbonate.

#85 Answer: A) *Down syndrome*

> *Williams syndrome* = cardiac defects (specifically, aortic stenosis), mental delays, "elfin" facies
> *Sticklers syndrome* = hearing/vision loss, cleft palate
> *Turner syndrome* = one X chromosome, aortic coarctation, webbed neck, ovarian hypofunction, short stature, normal intelligence
> *Down syndrome* = trisomy 21, 20 – 30% will have duodenal atresia, multiple other common anomalies, including congenital heart defects
> (*Lerman 6th ed*)

#86 Answer: B) *Free air under the diaphragm*

> Free air under the diaphragm indicates a bowel perforation, this is a possible outcome if necrotizing enterocolitis is not caught in time, or even if treated medically can still progress to perforation.

#87 Answer: A) *Double bubble sign*

> Duodenal atresia, double bubble on abdominal film represents air in enlarged stomach and proximal duodenum, with no air distal to duodenum; these patients have bilious vomiting as opposed to pyloric stenosis which is considered non-bilious vomiting

#88 Answer: C) *Intestines above the diaphragm*

Congenital diaphragmatic hernia patients have an incomplete fusion of the diaphragm; there is a defect, a hole, in the diaphragm that allows intestines, sometimes stomach, or even liver to herniate into the chest cavity. The presence of these organs in the chest is the cause of the lung hypoplasia, and resultant morbidity and mortality.

#89 Answer: D) *Olive-shaped mass*

The pylorus is the muscular valve connecting the stomach to the duodenum. In pyloric stenosis, this valve becomes hypertrophied, creating obstruction. It can be palpated in the upper left corner of the abdomen. It has been called "olive-shaped", due to its size and shape. Ultrasound is used for confirmation of diagnosis.

#90 Answer: C) *Male*

African Americans are 4 – 6X more likely to have OSA. Down syndrome patients have macroglossia and are predisposed and anticipated to have OSA. Obesity is clearly a risk factor for OSA. There are no gender predispositions for OSA. (*Cote 4th ed, p 661*)

#91 Answer: D) *Pinpoint pupils*

Apnea, dilated pupils and loss of consciousness are clinical signs of a high spinal. Recall the mechanism of a high spinal is local anesthetic at the level of the brain stem. Cranial nerve reflexes are abolished so the patient will lose consciousness, breathing will stop, and eye exam will reveal fixed, dilated pupils. Care is supportive; secure the airway. All spinal medications have a half-life so effects will fade with time.

#92 Answer: C) *368 ml*

First calculate patient's hourly fluid maintenance: 4-2-1 rule
For this 13 kg patient,

10 kg: 1st 10 kg	→ 4ml/hr × 10kg	= 40 ml/hr
3 kg: 2nd 10 – 20 kg	→ 2 ml/hr × 3 kg	= 6 ml/hr
0 kg: additional kgs	→ 1ml/hr × 0 kg	= 0 ml/hr
	Total	= 46 ml/hr.

For deficit of 8 hours, multiply maintenance ml/hr × NPO hr
46 ml/ hr × 8 hr = 368 ml total deficit

#93 Answer: A) *Ketamine*

Ketamine is still the gold standard induction drug for tetralogy of Fallot. Sevoflurane would be a bad choice as an induction agent, as an infant with congenital heart disease would potentially have profound cardiac compromise from a high forced inspired concentration of volatile anesthetic; even a low concentration of volatile agent can have deleterious cardiac effects. Propofol would not be ideal secondary to its potential to drop systemic vascular resistance; recall that maintaining or even increasing SVR is a goal in patients with TOF. Morphine is not an ideal induction agent for a 2-month-old patient. High dose narcotics are certainly a possibility for induction of a patient with congenital heart disease; fentanyl would be a preferred option if choosing a high dose narcotic induction. If you chose the latter option - high dose narcotic induction - extubating your patient at the end of a one hour case would be ill-advised, and quite possibly dangerous.

#94 Answer: B) *Ketamine*

The patient described has a pericardial effusion with signs and symptoms of tamponade. In addition to tachypnea, possible hypotension, you may see respiratory variation called "pulsus paradoxus" = greater than 10 mmHg decrease in systolic blood pressure during inspiration; normal respiratory variation is < 5 mmHg decrease in systolic blood pressure. The recommended induction agent in this scenario would be ketamine. Recall goals for tamponade: "full, fast, and tight". Cardiac output is dependent on: heart rate and stroke volume (CO = HR × SV). The stroke volume is considered "fixed" in this situation; the heart cannot expand to allow for increased stroke volume due to compression from fluid surrounding the heart. You want to augment preload as much as possible, by increasing intravascular volume (blood, NSS), keep the heart rate high, stroke volume "fixed" so cardiac output is relying on heart rate, and lastly tight=keep systemic vascular resistance (SVR) high. If you significantly decrease the SVR, the patient will have no preload or volume returning to their collapsed right atrium/ right ventricle, empty heart… boom…arrest. Opioids (morphine, fentanyl) can lower heart rate, and even SVR; sevoflurane decreases SVR; propofol can profoundly decrease SVR. Morphine, propofol and sevoflurane would not be considered ideal choices in this clinical scenario.

#95 Answer: D) *Prepare to shock*

The scenario describes a patient in cardiac arrest with pulseless ventricular tachycardia. The pediatric advance life support algorithm starts with: calling for help, get the code cart in the room, initiate chest compression, turn off volatile agent, deliver 100% oxygen, prepare to shock as soon as possible, alternating shocks with intravenous epinephrine every 3 – 5 min, after three shocks consider amiodarone, continue good quality chest compressions (presence of $ETCO_2$) until return of spontaneous, perfusing rhythm.

#96 Answer: B) *30 joules*

2 joules/kg is the correct calculation for initial shock, 4 joules/kg should be used if first shock is unsuccessful and repeat shock required.

#97 Answer: C) *Increased T waves*

Of the listed answers - increased HR greater than 10 beats/min, increased systolic blood pressure, and increased T waves – are all considered a positive test dose. The T wave changes will usually happen within 10 seconds of injection. Heart rate changes will follow shortly after the T waves changes. The T waves become very spiked and appear similar to hyperkalemia T waves; if you see this, remove your needle. If you have any signs of a positive test dose, remove your needle. If you see premature ventricular contractions in a patient that just received a block with local anesthetic, and this patient did not have PVCs prior to the block, this a precursor to possible cardiac toxicity. Prepare for possible cardiovascular collapse, pediatric advance life support algorithm, with intralipid available for this specific scenario, in addition to chest compressions, defibrillating pads, epinephrine etc.

#98 Answer: B) *False*

Normal resting ICP for a child is 2 – 4 mmHg, vs and adult is 10 – 15 mmHg. *(Cote 4th ed, p 511)*

#99 Answer: D) *Total lung capacity (ml/kg)*

Most of the lung volumes are the same in infants and adults on an ml/kg basis. The absolute values are less in infant. Total lung capacity however is less on an ml/kg basis in infants (63 ml/kg) compared to adults (82 ml/kg). *(Cote 4th ed, p 15)*

#100 Answer: B) *Inspiratory reserve volume*

As mention in previous answer, total lung capacity is reduced in infants. The two volumes that are considered "effort dependent" are inspiratory reserve volume and expiratory reserve volume. Inspiratory reserve volume is considerably decreased in infants and is the primary explanation for decreased total lung volume in infants. Closing Volumes and Residual Volumes are actually increased in infants. Closing volume does not actually have anything to do with total lung volumes. Closing volume is the lung volume at which the dependent regions of the lung start to "close" and atelectasis occurs. In infants, closing volume is usually within their normal tidal volume, in other words during normal tidal volume breathing they can develop atelectasis easily during normal expiration (lung volume decreased).

#101 Answer: D) *Unroasted peanut*

The unroasted peanut has greater potential for severe response because of the oils present. All airway foreign bodies are considered an emergency and should be removed. Timing of the removal involves discussion with ENT surgeon and the patient's clinical condition.

#102 Answer: A) *HR has greatest impact on cardiac output*

This is an important concept to understanding the hemodynamics of neonates. Due to the relatively stiff left ventricle, the neonate is reliant on heart rate to increase cardiac output. (*Cote 4th ed, p 324*)

#103 Answer: C) 142 mL

Estimated blood volume (EBV) in ml/kg:
- Premature neonates: 95 – 100 ml/kg
- Full term neonates: 85 ml/kg
- Infants: 80 ml/kg

EBV calculation: body wt (kg) × average blood volume (ml/kg)
    1.5 kg premature neonate × 95 ml/kg = 142.5 ml
These numbers vary slightly depending on source. (*Cote 4th ed, p 198-200*)

#104 Answer: C) *Hypoglycemia*

Glucose is the source of carbohydrates used in total parenteral nutrition (TPN). In the premature infant, glucose regulation may be challenging with the patient at risk for hypo- and hyperglycemic episodes. Glucose is the primary energy substrate for the brain, which makes up a greater proportion of body weight in preterm infants compared with term infants and older children. This results in a higher glucose metabolic requirement in premature infants. Hypoglycemia in an infant is considered <40 mg/dL, symptoms include jitteriness, convulsions, and apnea which may be difficult to appreciate in a patient under general anesthesia. (*Lerman 6th ed, p 33*)

#105 Answer: D) Increased, unchanged, and increased

Neonatal oxygen consumption (per kg) is 2 – 3 times that of the adult. Infant tidal volume is actually the same as adults (5 – 7 cc/kg), it is their high alveolar ventilation (RR), and high cardiac output (HR) that sustains a high VO_2. (*Cote 5th ed, p 358*).

#106 Answer: B) *2.5*

The correct endotracheal tube (ETT) size and length of insertion (tip to lip distance) can be estimated from the infant's weight. Depth is easily remembered as "1-2-3, 7-8-9."
1 kg - 2.5 ETT / 7 cm at lip
2 kg - 3.0 ETT / 8 cm at lip
3 kg - 3.5 ETT / 9 cm at lip
    Another formula: Insertion Depth (cm) = 6 + weight (kg)

(*Cote 4ed, p 252*)

#107 Answer: C) *Intubate the trachea*

Early intubation and gastric decompression is essential in patients with congenital diaphragmatic hernias. Positive pressure ventilation with facemask is very risky because the lungs are noncompliant and distension of the stomach and intestines can further compress the thoracic contents. This patient is clearly in distress based on the clinical presentation and vital signs provided. Intubation should take place promptly. Goals for congenital diaphragmatic hernia include, permissive hypercapnea = low tidal volumes. Pulmonary hypertension will determine patient's risk for morbidity and mortality. Inhaled nitric oxide, in addition to extracorporeal membrane oxygenation, has been used routinely to stabilize these patients. (*Cote 4th p 286*) (*Smith's 7th edition, p.547-549*)

#108 Answer: A) Increased O_2 consumption

Neonates have a very high metabolic oxygen consumption compared to adults (6 – 8 ml/kg/min vs 3 – 4 ml/kg/min). It does not matter how long you pre-oxygenate a one-week-old infant because once you stop ventilation they will begin to desaturate within 60 seconds. Functional residual capacity is the same on ml/kg basis, and total lung capacity is reduced in a neonate.

#109 Answer: D) *Succinylcholine*

All inhalation anesthetics except nitrous oxide are triggers for malignant hyperthermia (MH). Succinylcholine, the only depolarizing muscle relaxant, is also a trigger for malignant hyperthermia. No other anesthetic drugs appear to be triggers. (*Cote 4th ed, p 110,129*)

#110 Answer: B) *Elevated temperature*

The earliest signs are rise in end-expired carbon dioxide concentration despite increased minute ventilation, tachycardia, tachypnea, accompanied by muscle rigidity, especially following succinylcholine administration. Body temperature elevation is a dramatic but often late sign of MH (*Cote 5th ed, p 818-820*)

#111 Answer: D) *Discontinue triggering agent*

Immediately discontinue any triggering agents: inhalational anesthetics, succinylcholine. If possible end surgery, life-threatening surgery can be continued, but with the use of a non-triggering anesthetic agent (propofol infusion). Call for help, 100% oxygen, hyperventilate patient, and initiate treatment with dantrolene, in addition to actively cooling patient. Patient may require sodium bicarbonate for severe acidosis, calcium or insulin glucose or face life-threatening hyperkalemia. *MHAUS.org*

#112 Answer: A) *Cryoprecipitate*

Cryoprecipitate contains approximately 200 mg of fibrinogen and 100 units of factor VIII, 4 – 8 times that of FFP. (*Cote 5th ed, p 416*)

#113 Answer: A) *Factor VII*

150 – 250 ml of fibrinogen, contains
- 80 – 100 units of Factor VIII
- Von Willebrand factor
- Factor XIII
- Fibronectin

(*Cote 5th ed, p 415-418*)

#114 Answer: C) *Hemophilia A*

Cryoprecipitate contains fibrinogen and factor VIII (see answer #112). Hemophilia A is a bleeding disorder caused by deficiency of clotting factor VIII. Hemophilia B is caused by a deficiency or dysfunction of factor IX resulting from a variety of defects in the factor IX gene. (*Cote 5th ed, p 191-192*)

#115 Answer: D) *Umbilical artery - Hypogastric artery - Common Iliac artery - Aorta*

The umbilical artery carries deoxygenated blood from the fetus to the placenta. The path of an umbilical artery catheter starts at the umbilical artery, travels through the hypogastric artery to the common iliac artery and into the aorta. (*Cote 4th ed, p 1061*)

#116 Answer: A) *Choanal atresia*

Infants are preferential nose breathers; choanal atresia is a blocked nasal passage, usually due to narrowing of the nasal cavity. It can be unilateral or bilateral, it is very rare, and occurs in females > males. If the nasal passages are blocked the infant may become cyanotic at rest, but when crying the infant breaths through the mouth, air reaches the lungs, cyanosis is reduced or eliminated. (*uptodate*)

#117 Answer: B) *Increase inspiratory time*

As we age, our respiratory rate decreases and tidal volumes increase. Inspiratory time increases as respiratory rate decreased to allow more time for inhalation. These ventilator adjustments should be made as a neonate grows if long term ventilator support is required. (*uptodate*)

#118 Answer: B) *Fetal hemoglobin*

> Left-shifted curve signifies less O_2 delivery to tissues due to higher affinity of oxygen to hemoglobin. Fetal hemoglobin, alkalosis, hypocarbia, and hypothermia result in a left shift of the oxy-hemoglobin curve. Right-shift allows more O_2 delivery to tissues due to decreased hemoglobin affinity for O_2. (*Cote 5th ed, p 770-771*)

#119 Answer: C) *Right hand and left foot*

> Remember, the ductus arteriosus connects the pulmonary artery to the arch/descending aorta. To obtain pre- and post-ductal oxygen saturations, you should place a pulse oximeter on the upper right extremity and one on the lower extremities. The left upper extremity is not utilized at it has traditionally been considered indeterminate; could be pre ductal, could be post ductal. The concern with the left hand is its blood supply, the left subclavian is extremely close to the juncture of the ductus arteriosus and the aorta, thus the left subclavian may have mixed blood if shunt exists across ductus. (*Cote 5th ed, p 354-356*)

#120 Answer: D) *Significant right-to-left shunt*

> A gradient of more than 10% between a pre- and post-ductal SpO_2 indicates a shunt significant enough to cause deoxygenated blood to be redirected via a communication i.e. the PDA to systemic circulation, or can result from a congenital cardiac anomaly. (*Cote 5th ed, p 361-362*)

#121 Answer: B) *Persistent pulmonary hypertension of the newborn*

> Persistent pulmonary hypertension of the newborn (PPHN) occurs when pulmonary vascular resistance (PVR) remains abnormally elevated after birth, resulting in right-to-left shunting of blood. The definitive diagnosis of (PPHN) is made by echocardiography. In PPHN, echocardiogram demonstrates normal structural cardiac anatomy with evidence of pulmonary hypertension. Persistent pulmonary hypertension of newborn has many possible etiologies: asphyxia, meconium aspiration, sepsis, stress. Other considerations for the pre and post-ductal gradient must be ruled out: congenital cardiac lesions! *(Cote 4th ed, p. 750)*

#122 Answer: D) *All of the above*

> Understanding the pathophysiology of pulmonary hypertension is crucial. When pulmonary vascular pressures are elevated, there are two possible mechanisms resulting in hypoxia: vasoconstriction of pulmonary vasculature which decreases pulmonary blood flow and shunting of blood where blood takes the path of least resistance and is redirected through the PDA and/or PFO. In order to correct this hypoxic mixture you must reverse the pressure gradient. The most potent pulmonary vasodilator is O_2, so 100% FiO_2 is initially used. Next, inhaled nitric oxide can be used to reduce pulmonary vascular resistance. The patients become dependent on preload as a way to maintain cardiac output. Lastly, increasing SVR with a vasopressor will help reverse a right-to-left shunt. (*Cote 5th ed, p 749*)

#123 Answer: B) *"Boot-shaped" heart on CXR*

#124 Answer: D) *Significant cardiomegaly, right aortic arch*

#125 Answer: C) *Figure of eight, "snowman" sign on CXR, normal heart size*

#126 Answer: A) *"Box-shaped" heart on CXR*

> **Tetralogy of Fallot** - four malformations include: ventricular septal defect, pulmonary stenosis, overriding aorta and right ventricular hypertrophy. Chest X-ray findings can include a boot-shaped heart.
> **Truncus arteriosus** - Involves an arterial trunk that originates from both ventricles of the heart that later divides into the aorta and the pulmonary trunk. Chest X-ray findings can reveal a right-sided aortic arch and significant cardiomegaly.
> **Total anomalous pulmonary venous return** - Involves all four pulmonary veins being malpositioned (pulmonary veins don't bring O_2-Hb back to left atrium). Chest X-ray shows the snowman sign or "figure of 8" configuration.
> **Ebstein anomaly** - the septal and posterior leaflets of the tricuspid valve are displaced towards the apex of the right ventricle of the heart. Chest X-ray shows a box-shaped heart.
> (*Cote 5th ed, p 291-294*)

#127 Answer: D) *A & B*

> Changing the frequency (Hertz), amplitude, and inspiratory time will all change the tidal volume and thus alter CO_2. (*Cote 5th ed, p 276*)

#128 Answer: C) *Hertz*

> The frequency setting is measured in Hertz (Hz). One Hertz is equal to 1 breath per second or 60 breaths per minute (e.g. 10 Hz = 600 breaths per minute). Changes in frequency are inversely proportional to the amplitude and thus delivered tidal volume. (*Cote 5th ed, p 276*)

#129 Answer: D) *Chest wiggle*

> Chest wiggle – rapid chest wall movement occurring with delivery of small volumes in HFOV - is often used clinically to evaluate for adequate lung expansion. (*uptodate*).

#130 Answer: D) *All of the above*

Protamine, if given rapidly or in excess, can lead to devastating consequences. All of the answers choices are potential side effects in addition to hemorrhagic pulmonary edema. In regards to the coagulation abnormalities, a protamine: heparin ratio in excess of 2.6:1 can lead to an increasing ACT, while platelet aggregation can occur with minimal excess protamine. (*Cote 5th ed, p 414*)

Protamine Reactions
Protamine is a naturally occurring protein (+) charge used to neutralize heparin (-) charge

HORROW CLASSIFICATION OF PROTAMINE REACTION
I. Hypotension: histamine, rapid administration
II. Anaphylaxis
    a. Anaphylaxis: **IgE**
    b. Immediate anaphylactoid: complement activation
    c. Delayed anaphylactioid: complement activation
III. Catastrophic pulmonary vasoconstriction
    Right ventricular failure, cardiovascular collapse, **thromboxane A2**

[Jay Horrow, MD was chairman during my anesthesiology residency at Drexel University School of Medicine/Hahnemann University Hospital. I have found this classification the most straightforward way to remember potential reactions. -ERB]

#131 Answer: B) *Good choice to augment contractility and perfusion, used in patients with compromised ventricular function or patients with anaphylaxis.*

Epi effects α and β receptors,+ chronotropy as well as inotropy, increased diastolic pressure (vasoconstriction), diminished splenic perfusion possible.

#132 Answer: F) *Selective beta 1 (minimal beta 2) activity with side effects including tachycardia and vasodilation.*

Dobutamine is used to increase cardiac output by increasing myocardial output.

#133 Answer: D) *Positive inotropy and lusitropy by increasing cyclic adenosine monophosphate (cAMP).*

Milrinone is considered a phosphodiesterase inhibitor, this increases cAMP which in turn increased intracellular Ca^{2+} level, may cause hypotension

#134 Answer: A) *Can increase splanchnic and renal perfusion even at high doses.*

Dopamine effects α, β, and DA receptors. Dopamine indirect effects are due to norepinephrine release.

#135 Answer: E) *Pure, nonselective beta agonist. May be useful in children with bradycardia or post-heart transplant patients as a pharmacological pacemaker.*

#136 Answer: C) *Increases SVR as a pure alpha agonist. Can cause significant reflex bradycardia.*

(Faust, p 194-198)

#137 Answer: D) *Inhaled nitric oxide*

Nitric oxide is used frequently for the treatment of pulmonary hypertension. It is delivered directly to the pulmonary circulation through inhalation. Nitric oxide is an endothelium-derived relaxing factor that acts on guanylate cyclase in vascular smooth muscle. It is bound rapidly in the blood by oxyhemoglobin which is then converted to methemoglobin. It is this reaction that overtime can lead to methemoglobinemia. *(Cote 5th ed, p 748)*

#138 Answer: A) *Antithrombin III deficiency*

Heparin produces anticoagulation by combining with antithrombin III (ATIII), which then binds to and inhibits thrombin. In patient with ATIII deficiency, heparin may not achieve adequate anticoagulation. Treatment in this circumstance includes recombinant ATIII or FFP to replace the ATIII. *(Cote 5th ed, p 390)*

#139 D) *100%*

An otherwise healthy infant's weight should double at six months of age. Birth weight should triple at one year. *(uptodate)*

#140 C) *60 cm H_2O*

A healthy term newborn can generate up to 40 – 60 cm H_2O negative pressure for their first breath. Consider the resistance to that first breath, as the lungs have never been fully expanded, and certainly not with air. The alveoli are filled with amniotic fluid and there is tremendous resistance to expand for the first time. *(Barash 7th ed, p 1180)*

#141 B) *Height*

#142 A) *Intramuscular*

Onset in this order, with *approximate* bioavailability in parenthesis: intravenous (1.0) > intramuscular (0.9) > intranasal (0.5) = sublingual (0.5) > rectal (0.4) >oral (0.3). Please note that bioavailability values, as with all numbers, vary slightly from source to source.

#143 D) *Sagittal*

Craniosynostosis is a premature closure of cranial sutures. Recall at birth an infant has several fontanelles, which represents non-union of the skull as specific suture lines. In order of frequency the list of premature closures are sagittal > coronal > metopic. Most patients with this anomaly are non-syndromic, healthy infants. *(Cote 4th ed, p 702)*

#144 Answer A) *Left ventricular end diastolic diameter*

Shortening fraction is an alternative method of estimating global cardiac function. It is calculated with ECHO using the following parameters:

$$\frac{\text{LV end diastolic diameter} - \text{LV end diastolic diameter}}{\text{LV end diastolic diameter}}$$

Normal shortening fraction = 30 – 40%
Normal ejection fraction (EF) >60%
EF = (SV - EDV) - 100

#145 Answer C) *Perimembranous*

In order of frequency, perimembranous (80%) > muscular (5 – 20%) > inlet (5 – 7%) > subarterial (5 – 7%) Recall that VSD is the most common congenital heart defect; incidence 1.5-3.5: 1000 live births. *(Lake 4th ed, p 337)*

#146 Answer D) *Pulmonary vascular congestion*

Recall a VSD is considered a left-to-right shunt, so typically these patients do not present with cyanosis. A left to right shunt, as with all shunts, depends on the balance between pulmonary vascular resistance (PVR) and systemic vascular resistance (SVR). As PVR decreases after birth, a large defect will allow increases in the blood shunted from the left to right ventricle, and result in over perfusion of the lungs, often resulting in CHF, frequent pulmonary infections, pulmonary hypertension, and failure to thrive secondary to poor feedings.

Increased hematocrit is a common finding in patients with cyanotic lesions. Hematocrit increases as a compensatory mechanism in responses to decrease oxygen saturation to increase delivery of oxygen (DO_2).

DO_2 = cardiac output × O_2 content [Hgb × 1.36 × SaO_2 + {0.0031 × PaO_2}]

#147 Answer C) *Lungs*

Many drugs have increased uptake and metabolism by the lungs, prostaglandins are on the list. Others include: opioids (fentanyl 90%, meperidine > 90%), lidocaine, norepinephrine (3-16%), dopamine, propranolol (70%), steroids (progesterone, beclomethasone), serotonin, bradykinin, and adenosine. *(Boer F. Drug Handling by The Lungs. British Journal of Anaestheisa. 2003; 91: 50-60)*

#148 Answer C) *160 beats/minute*

Let me say that as always when it comes to numbers, the answer ranges depend on what book you reference. As a very general rule, heart rate depends on age

- <1 yo   100 – 160 bpm   < 100 = bradycardia, > 200 tachycardia
- 1 – 2 yo   90 – 140 bpm
- 2 – 5 yo   80 – 140 bpm
- 6 – 12 yo   70 – 120

Almost all human beings will have decreased heart rate with sleep.

#149 Answer C) *Increased, decreased, increased*

Onset of muscle relaxant is increased in a neonate. Decreased clearance of rocuronium is expected in neonates (diminished liver / renal function). Potency of muscle relaxant is dramatically increased in neonates> adults> infant

#150 Answer B) *"Machine-like"*

The murmur description for a patent ductus arteriosus is often reported to be a continuous, machine-like sound. Recall that blood will flow through a PDA during systole and diastole.
- Mill-wheel murmur = associated with a cardiac air embolism
- Austin-Flint = aortic insufficiency/regurgitation
    - Low-pitched rumbling murmur best heard at cardiac apex
- Still's Murmur = common pediatric finding, aka "innocent murmur"
    - Low-pitched with musical quality best heard at left sternal border

Aortic insufficiency (AI) and PDA have some similar qualities, both are considered to have diastolic runoff, AI- blood runoff back into LV during diastole, PDA- runoff back to lungs, both have widened pulse pressure (difference between systolic and diastolic pressure) you will see a low diastolic pressure (DP), both can have coronary artery perfusion compromise as a result of low diastolic pressure. LVEDP = left ventricular end-diastolic pressure

Coronary perfusion pressure = DP - LVEDP

#151 Answer D) *Umbilical vein*

Recall the umbilical vein brings oxygenated blood from the placenta to the fetus, it carries the highest PaO_2 and oxygen saturation in fetal circulation, this blood will empty into the IVC. Once blood reaches the right atrium it has begun to be mixed with systemic de-oxygenated blood returning to the heart, and will naturally begin to have a decreased oxygen saturation and partial pressure.

Approximate oxygen saturations in utero:
- Umbilical vein: 70%
- IVC: 70%
- Right atrium: 55%
- Left atrium: 65%
- Pulmonary artery: 55%
- Ductus arteriosus: 55%
- Umbilical artery: 45%

The left atrium is slightly higher than the right atrium, because the oxygenated blood (70%) from the IVC is preferentially shunted via the foramen ovale from the right atrium to the left atrium. (*Cote 4th ed, p 363*)

#152 Answer A) *Decreased oxygen binding*

Hemoglobin F has a left-shifted oxygen-hemoglobin dissociation curve, with a p50 of approximately 19 mmHg, this represents INCREASED oxygen binding to the heme molecule. A p50 of 19 mmHg means less partial pressure of oxygen is required to have 50% of the heme saturated. Hemoglobin F, increased hematocrit, increased 2,3-DPG and increased cardiac output all help with oxygen delivery to the fetal vital organs and uptake at the level of the placenta.

#153 Answer C) *Pediatric patients have increased risk for morbidity and mortality*

Pediatric patients have increased risk for morbidity and mortality with regards to anesthesia. This has been documented in numerous studies. The highest risk patients for general anesthesia are neonates and children less than one year of age. Morbidity is 35% of all pediatric cases vs 17% for adults. (*Anesthesia Related Cardiac Arrest in children, Initial findings of the pediatric perioperative cardiac arrest registry (POCA) Morray JP. Anesthesiology. 2000, July: 93 (1): 6-14) (Cohen MM. 1990. Pediatric Anesthesia morbidity and mortality in perioperative period. Anesthesia and Analgesia. Feb 70 (2), p 160-67*)

#154 Answer A) *19 mmHg*

Hb A p50= 26 mmHg, Hb SS p50= 30 mmHg

#155 Answer A) *Decreased protein concentration*

Plasma protein binding determines cardiovascular risks. Free-unbound (i.e. active) drug produces toxicity. Neonates naturally have decreased protein concentration; therefore, they have a higher percentage of unbound free drug. Neonates do, in fact, also have a higher cardiac output, which increases delivery of drug to organs, and they also have an increased percentage of cardiac output to the vessel rich organs (brain, heart), so this too contributes to their increased risks. However decreased protein concentration is considered number one. The blood brain barrier (BBB) is considered by most resources as "immature" at birth, or not completely developed, implying its functional properties, i.e. limiting substances delivery/ penetration to the brain, may not be totally evolved. The BBB is often referred to as "leaky" in the newborn. There have been recent studies questioning this long held belief. Another way to think about this… almost all of the CNS continues to develop following birth: the brain, the skull, the sympathetic/parasympathetic, the neurons (myelination)… why wouldn't the blood brain barrier? With an immature BBB, I believe the general thought is you have increased delivery of drugs across to the brain, so this too would contribute to an increase in risks of local anesthetic toxicity or drugs in general in the newborn. (*Cote 4th ed, p 870*)

#156 Answer B) *2 – 6 mmHg*

2 – 6 mmHg is considered normal intracranial pressure for a neonate. Less than 15 mmHg is considered normal for adults. (*Cote 4th ed, p 511*)

#157 Answer C) *2-year-old*

Age determines blood flow rates, these values are considered approximate for otherwise healthy patients.

Neonate/preterm infants	~ 40ml/100g/min
Children	~ 100ml/100g/min
Adult	~ 50ml/100g/min

(*Cote 4th ed, p 511*)

#158 Answer B) *pKa*

#159 Answer C) *Protein binding*

#160 Answer A) *Lipid solubility*

pKa - or dissociation constant: involves a logarithm calculation, the pKa number represents the pH at which the local anesthetic will exist as a mixture; 50% ionized form (charged), and 50% anionic form (uncharged = neutral) form. Recall the neutral form is lipid soluble and responsible for the amount of drug that penetrates the neural membrane. The more drug that penetrates the membrane the quicker the onset. Of note, the closer the pKa number is to physiologic pH 7.4, the more rapid the onset.
- *Compare: lidocaine pKa 7.9 vs bupivacaine pKa 8.1, lidocaine > bupivacaine onset.*

Protein binding: traditionally related to duration of action. Recall protein bound drug is considered "inactive", and free drug, non-bound drug is active. Increased protein binding = increases duration of action.
- *Compare: lidocaine 44% protein bound vs bupivacaine 95% protein bound, bupivacaine>>>lidocaine duration of action.*

Potency: as with most other drugs is related to lipid solubility, increased solubility = increased potency

#161 Answer C) *Perfusion*

During cardiopulmonary bypass hypothermia is induced and as the patient's blood cools, viscosity increases.
Do you remember the formula for resistance (R)?

$$R \alpha \frac{n \times L}{r^4}$$

n = viscosity, so as viscosity increases so too does resistance, if we decrease viscosity (lower hematocrit) we lower resistance and therefore improve perfusion.
L = length
r^4 = radius

#162 Answer C) *Down syndrome*

It is fair to say you could potentially see bradycardia during all of the above patients with an inhalation mask induction. And it is almost always true that after our patients have progressed through stage 2 of anesthesia their heart rates will decrease naturally. With a Down syndrome patient you should anticipate and prepare for possible profound bradycardia during a mask inhalation induction. You should first turn off the volatile agent, or at least significantly reduce the concentration as soon as the heart rate starts to drop. Secondly, prepare to give atropine either intravenous, or intramuscular if no IV obtained yet. The bradycardia is usually rapid, and dramatic, though it can be self-limiting once volatile agent removed. However it can and has resulted in cardiac arrest, so be aware. Forewarned is forearmed. *(Barash 7th ed, p 1245)*

#163 Answer D) *Gamma subunit*

Both fetal and adult neuromuscular junctions have five subunits; the fetal NMJ has a gamma subunit instead of the epsilon subunit found in the adult NMJ. Recall that the neuromuscular blocking agents attach to the alpha subunits, presents in both fetal and adult NMJ.

#164 Answer D) *10 years old*

Believe it or not the package insert for etomidate reads "There are inadequate data to make dosage requirements for induction of anesthesia in patients less than 10 years old; therefore such use in not recommended". That being said, I am aware that etomidate is used, though not frequently in pediatric patients less than ten years old, with the same dosing as for adults.

#165 Answer A) *2 months old*

Potency of neuromuscular relaxants is expected to be increased in infants less than one year old. A two-year-old and a ten-year-old should have the same expected onset and duration of action, assuming healthy patients. It is strongly recommended that that all neuromuscular relaxants should be completely reversed in infants regardless of duration of procedure if the time of the last dose is less than 2 hours. *(Barash 7th ed, p 1227)*

#166 Answer C) *Tissue: gas solubility*

Respiratory rate is dramatically increased in neonates (30 – 60 per minute) vs adults (12 – 16 per minute). Increased respiratory rate is the primary explanation for increased alveolar ventilation. Dead space in neonates and adults should be the same on an mL/kg basis. Oxygen consumption is increased in neonates (6 – 8 ml/kg/min) vs adults (3 – 4 ml/kg/min). Blood: gas solubility is decreased in neonates, by as much as 18%. Recall decreased blood: gas solubility increases wash in effect (onset). The decreased solubility is thought to be secondary to increased volume of distribution, as well as diminished circulating proteins. *(Cote 4th ed, p 103)*

167 Answer B) *6 – 12 months*

> Separation anxiety is a completely normal development in infants, it is considered a milestone. Typically presents anytime between the ages of 6 – 12 months. It represents a time in the infants life when they become aware of who their daily caregivers are, and everyone who isn't! Separation can cause great distress in infants, which will generally results in crying.

#168 Answer C) *Intubate and suction meconium contents from lungs*

> In a child with low APGAR scores or an infant in distress, the infant's oro- and nasopharynx should be immediately suctioned followed by endotracheal intubation and suctioning of any meconium that is present below the cords. In a clinically well-appearing, vigorously crying newborn without meconium at the level of the vocal cords, intubation may not be necessary. (*Cote 5th ed, p 17*)

#169 Answer: D) *Predominately dilates venous capacitance vessels by smooth muscle relaxation.*

#170 Answer: A) *Dilates both arterial and venous capacitance vessels. reflex tachycardia in addition to cyanide toxicity are possible side effects.*

#171 Answer: E) *Selective alpha receptor blocker, greatest activity on arterial vessels.*

#172 Answer: B) *Direct acting smooth muscle dilator with a long duration of action. Can cause lupus-like syndrome, drug fever, and thrombocytopenia.*

#173 Answer: C) *Direct smooth muscle relaxation, can cause apnea in neonates.*

#174 Answer: F) *Short acting beta blocker (beta 1 selective). Rapid onset/offset. (Faust. 3rd Edition p 199-205)*

175 Answer A) *Ear*

> Desaturation response times range from 7.2 – 19.8 seconds for ear probes, from 19.5 – 35.1 for finger probes and from 41.0 – 72.6 seconds for toe probes. Thus the most accurate site in terms of limiting delay in pulse oximetry reading is the ear. (*Faust's 3rd Edition p 31*)

176 Answer B) *Vasopressin*

The mnemonic **LEAN** is an easy way to remember the emergency medications that can be administered via endotracheal tube (ETT) in pediatrics:
Lidocaine, **E**pinephrine, **A**tropine, **N**aloxone.
According to American Heart Association Guidelines:
- **Vasopressin** - There is no current recommendation for use of vasopressin in pediatric patients.
- **Epinephrine** - pediatric endotrachial dose of epinephrine be increased by approximately 10 times the standard **intravenous dose of 0.1 mL/kg of a 1:10 000 solution (0.01 mg/kg) ETT dose = 1 mL/kg of 1:10 000 solution or 0.1 mg/kg).** For neonatal resuscitation, ETT doses of epinephrine up to 0.1 mg/kg of a 1 to 10 000 (0.1 mg/mL) are suggested.
- **Atropine** - pediatric ET dose should be 0.04 to 0.6 mg/kg with a minimal dose of 0.1 mg.
- **Naloxone** - not recommended for endotracheal use in neonates; for pediatric patients, the AHA states that other routes are preferred.

#177 Answer B) *Sevoflurane*

Hyperventilation, head up, mannitol and steroids have been shown to decrease intracranial pressure (ICP). Hyperventilation decreases ICP through cerebral vasoconstriction. Mannitol decrease cerebral blood volume by reducing cerebral parenchymal cell water. Steroids can decrease ICP through reduction in cerebral edema in patients with an intracranial mass (not indicated in traumatic brain injuries). All inhalational anesthetics increase ICP through vasodilation and increased cerebral perfusion. (*Cote 5ed, p 510-512*)

#178 Answer A) *2.5 ml/kg*

#179 Answer C) *30 ml/kg*

#180 Answer B) *7 ml/kg*

#181 Answer E) *82 ml/kg*

#182 Answer D) *63 ml/kg*

#183 Answer B) Prolonged QT interval

Peaked T waves are associated with hyperkalemia, and a positive test dose with local anesthetic. **U waves** follow the T wave on ECG, many etiologies but—most commonly—bradycardia, and severe hypokalemia. **J waves** (Osborn waves) also have many etiologies including hypothermia as well as severe head injury.

The Authors would like to thank the following:

Daniel Corn MD, John Crowe, MD, Alberto de Armendi MD, Cassandra Duncan-Azadi MD, James Eiszner MD, Andrew Fine MD, Judith Handley MD, Eric Holland APRN, CRNA, Sri Smitha Kanaparthy MD, Carol Loeber APRN-CNP, Evangelyn Okereke, MD, Nathan Overbey MD, Kamilah Shy MD, and Lauren Sparks MD

Chapter 14: Sources Consulted/ References

Andropoulos D et al. 2010. Anesthesia for Congenital Heart Disease (2nd Edition). Chichester: Blackwell Publishing Ltd.

ASA, 2011 Practice Guideline for preoperative fasting and the use of pharmacologic agents to reduce risk of pulmonary aspiration. Anesthesiology 114 (3), p 495-511.

Barash P et al. 2009 Clinical Anesthesia (6th Edition), Philadelphia, Lippincott Williams & Wilkins.

Barash P et al. 2013 Clinical Anesthesia (7th Edition). Philadelphia: Lippincott Williams & Wilkins.

Baugh R et al. 2011. Clinical Practice Guideline: Tonsillectomy in Children. Otolaryngology-Head and Neck Surgery 144(1), S 1-30.

Bhanaker,S et al. 2007. Anesthesia-Related Cardiac Arrest in Children: Update from the Pediatric Perioperative Cardiac Arrest Registry. International Anesthesia Research Society 105 (2), 344-350.

Boer F. 2003. Drug Handling by The Lungs. British Journal of Anaetheisa. 91: 50-60

Butterworth JF, Mackey DC, Wasnick JD. 2013. Morgan & Mikhail's Clinical Anesthesia (5th Edition). New York: McGraw-Hill Companies Inc.

Brennan,K, MD. 2016. Assessment and Management of a patient for the EXIT procedure. Anesthesiology News, 42 (2), 31-34.

cdc.gov

Codeine: Drug Information Lexicomp. UpToDate, 2015.

Cohen MM. 1990. Pediatric Anesthesia morbidity and mortality in perioperative period. Anesthesia and Analgesia. Feb 70 (2), p 160-67.

Cote CJ, et al, editors.2013. A Practice of Anesthesia for Infants and Children (5th ed), Philadelphia , Elsevier Saunders..

Cote CJ. 1995. Postoperative apnea in former preterm infants after inguinal herniorrhaphy. A combined analysis. Anesthesiology 82 (4), p 809-22.

Cote CJ, Lerman J, Todres.D. A Practice of Anesthesia For Infants and Children (4th Edition). Philadelphia: Elsevier, 2009.

Drug Package Inserts:
  Ketorolac- Hospira
  Succinylcholine- Hospira
  Precedex- Hospira

Dunn L. 2002. Raised Intracranial Pressure. Neurology Neurosurg Psychiatry 73 (1), p 23-27.

Dutoit A. 2015. Pediatric Anesthesia Pocket Reference Card, The Children's Hospital at OU Medical Center.

Faust RJ, et al, editors. 2001. Faust Anesthesiology Review (3rd Edition), New York, Churchill Livingstone.

fda.gov

Gregory G. 2002. Pediatric Anesthesia (4th Edition). Philadelphia: Churchill Livingstone.

Harden RN, Bruehl S, Perez RSGM, et al. 2010. Validation of proposed diagnostic criteria (the "Budapest Criteria") for Complex Regional Pain Syndrome. Pain. 150(2):268-274.

Kleinman M. et al "Part 14: Pediatric Advanced Life Support: 2010 American Heart Association Guidelines for Cardiopulmonary Resuscitation and Emergency Cardiovascular Care." Circulation 122.18, suppl 3.

Lake, Carol. 2005. Pediatric Cardiac Anesthesia (4th Edition). Philadelphia: Lippincott Williams & Wilkins.

Lerman J, Cote CJ. Steward DJ. 2010. Manual of Pediatric Anesthesia (6th edition). Philadelphia: Churchill Livingstone Elsevier.

mhaus.org, Malignant Hyperthermia Association of the United States

Miller RD et al, editors. 2005. Basics of Anesthesia (6th Edition), New York, Churchill Livingstone.

Morray J et al. 2000. Anesthesia-related Cardiac Arrest in Children. Anesthesiology 93 (6), 6-14.

Motoyama EK, Davis PJ. 2006. Smith's Anesthesia for Infants and Children (7th edition). Philadelphia, Elsevier.

Somerville N and Fenlon S. 2005. Anaesthesia for cleft lip and palate surgery. Continuing Ed in Anaesthesia, Critical care and pain 5 (3), 76-79.

Subramanyam R and Chung F. 2010. Perioperative Management of Obstructive Sleep Apnea Patients. Medicamundi 54.3 (2010): 41-46.

Vlajkovic GP, Sindjelic RP. 2006. Emergence Delirium in Children: Many Questions, Few Answers. International Anesthesia Research Society 104 (1), p 84-91.

www.heart.org 2010 American Heart Association Guidelines, Pediatric Advance Life support/ Neonatal resuscitation

Made in the USA
Middletown, DE
14 January 2018